Acute and Reconstructive Burn Care, Part I

Editors

FRANCESCO M. EGRO
C. SCOTT HULTMAN

CLINICS IN
PLASTIC SURGERY

www.plasticsurgery.theclinics.com

April 2024 • Volume 51 • Number 2

ELSEVIER

1600 John F. Kennedy Boulevard ● Suite 1800 ● Philadelphia, Pennsylvania, 19103-2899

http://www.theclinics.com

CLINICS IN PLASTIC SURGERY Volume 51, Number 2
April 2024 ISSN 0094-1298, ISBN-13: 978-0-443-13065-6

Editor: Stacy Eastman
Developmental Editor: Anita Chamoli

Clinics in Plastic Surgery (ISSN 0094-1298) is published quarterly by Elsevier Inc., 360 Park Avenue South, New York, NY 10010-1710. Months of issue are January, April, July, and October. Business and Editorial Offices: 1600 John F. Kennedy Blvd., Suite 1800, Philadelphia, PA 19103-2899. Periodicals postage paid at New York, NY and additional mailing offices. Subscription prices are $576.00 per year for US individuals, $100.00 per year for US students/residents, $631.00 per year for Canadian individuals, $703.00 per year for international individuals, $100.00 per year for Canadian students/residents, and $305.00 per year for international students/residents. For institutional access pricing please contact Customer Service via the contact information below. To receive student/resident rate, orders must be accompanied by name of affiliated institution, date of term, and the *signature* of program/residency coordinator on institution letterhead. Orders will be billed at individual rate until proof of status is received. Foreign air speed delivery is included in all *Clinics* subscription prices. All prices are subject to change without notice. **POSTMASTER:** Send address changes to *Clinics in Plastic Surgery*, Elsevier Health Sciences Division, Subscription Customer Service, 3251 Riverport Lane, Maryland Heights, MO 63043. **Customer Service: 1-800-654-2452 (US and Canada). From outside of the United States and Canada, call 314-447-8871. Fax: 314-447-8029. E-mail: JournalsCustomerService-usa@elsevier.com (for print support); JournalsOnlineSupport-usa@elsevier.com (for online support).**

Reprints. For copies of 100 or more of articles in this publication, please contact the Commercial Reprints Department, Elsevier Inc., 360 Park Avenue South, New York, New York 10010-1710. Tel.: +1-212-633-3874; Fax: +1-212-633-3820; E-mail: reprints@elsevier.com.

Clinics in Plastic Surgery is covered in *Current Contents, EMBASE/Excerpta Medica, Science Citation Index, MEDLINE/ PubMed (Index Medicus), ASCA, and ISI/BIOMED.*

Contributors

EDITORS

FRANCESCO M. EGRO, MD, MSc, MRCS
Associate Professor Department of Plastic
Surgery, Associate Professor Department of
Surgery, Deputy Chief of Plastic Surgery
UPMC Mercy, Associate Director of UPMC
Mercy Burn Center, Director of Burn
Reconstruction, Director of Medical Student
Education, Associate Program Director
Integrated & Independent Residency,
University of Pittsburgh Medical Center,
Pittsburgh, Pennsylvania

C. SCOTT HULTMAN, MD, MBA, FACS
Director, WPP Plastic and Reconstructive
Surgery, WakeMed Health and Hospitals,
Raleigh, North Carolina; Professor of Surgery,
Campbell University, Buies Creek, North
Carolina; Adjunct Professor, Department of
Plastic and Reconstructive Surgery, The Johns
Hopkins University School of Medicine, Johns
Hopkins University, Baltimore, Maryland

AUTHORS

YASMIN ALI, MD, MPH
Assistant Professor, Trauma Surgery and
Critical Care, Department of Surgery, College
of Medicine, University of Tennessee Health
Science Center, Memphis, Tennessee

JESSICA BALLOU, MD
Burn and Surgical Critical Care Fellow, Johns
Hopkins Department of Plastic and
Reconstructive Surgery, Johns Hopkins Burn
Center, Baltimore, Maryland

MARTIN R. BUTA, MD, MBA
Clinical Research Fellow, Plastic,
Reconstructive, and Laser Surgery, Shriners
Hospitals for Children, Tampa, Florida; Division
of Plastic and Reconstructive Surgery,
Massachusetts General Hospital, Harvard
Medical School, Boston, Massachusetts

AUDRA T. CLARK, MD
Assistant Professor, UT Southwestern Division of
Burn, Trauma, Acute and Critical Care Surgery,
UT Southwestern Medical Center, Dallas, Texas

ZACHARY J. COLLIER, MD, MS
Division of Plastic and Reconstructive Surgery,
USC Department of Surgery, University of
Chicago, Los Angeles, California

ALAIN C. CORCOS, MD, FACS
Associate Professor, Medical Director, Division
of Multisystem Trauma, Department of
Surgery, University of Pittsburgh Medical
Center, UPMC Mercy Hospital, Pittsburgh,
Pennsylvania

MATTHIAS B. DONELAN, MD
Chief of Staff, Plastic, Reconstructive, and
Laser Surgery, Shriners Hospitals for Children,
Tampa, Florida; Division of Plastic and
Reconstructive Surgery, Massachusetts
General Hospital, Harvard Medical School,
Boston, Massachusetts

FRANCESCO M. EGRO, MD, MSc, MRCS
Associate Professor Department of Plastic
Surgery, Associate Professor Department of
Surgery, Deputy Chief of Plastic Surgery
UPMC Mercy, Associate Director of UPMC
Mercy Burn Center, Director of Burn
Reconstruction, Director of Medical Student
Education, Associate Program Director
Integrated & Independent Residency,
University of Pittsburgh Medical Center,
Pittsburgh, Pennsylvania

JONATHAN FRIEDSTAT, MD, MPH, FACS
Acute Burn and Reconstructive Plastic
Surgeon, Department of Surgery,
Massachusetts General Hospital Shriner's
Hospital for Children - Boston; Assistant
Professor of Surgery, Harvard Medical School,
Boston, Massachusetts

JUSTIN GILLENWATER, MD, MS
Assistant Professor, Medical Director,
Department of Plastic and Reconstructive
Surgery, University of Southern California, Los
Angeles, California

POOJA GUPTA, MD
Associate Professor, Department of Pulmonary
and Critical Care, University of Tennessee
Health Science Center, Memphis, Tennessee

**DAVID M. HILL, PharmD, BCPS, BCCCP,
FCCM**
Associate Professor, Department of Pharmacy,
Regional One Health, University of Tennessee,
Memphis, Tennessee

C. SCOTT HULTMAN, MD, MBA, FACS
Director, WPP Plastic and Reconstructive
Surgery, WakeMed Health and Hospitals,
Raleigh, North Carolina; Professor of Surgery,
Campbell University, Buies Creek, North
Carolina; Adjunct Professor, Department of
Plastic and Reconstructive Surgery, The Johns
Hopkins University School of Medicine, Johns
Hopkins University, Baltimore, Maryland

ELIZABETH M. KENNY, MD
Resident Physician, Department of Plastic
Surgery, University of Pittsburgh Medical
Center, Pittsburgh, Pennsylvania

KEVIN M. KLIFTO, DO, PharmD
Resident Physician, Division of Plastic and
Reconstructive Surgery, Department of
Surgery, University of Missouri School of
Medicine, Columbia, Missouri

TOMER LAGZIEL, MD
Resident Physician, Department of Plastic and
Reconstructive Surgery, The Johns Hopkins
University School of Medicine, Baltimore,
Maryland

JULIO LANFRANCO, MD, MPH
Associate Professor, Chief, Division of
Pulmonary and Critical Care, University of

Tennessee Health Science Center, Memphis,
Tennessee

HAKAN ORBAY, MD, PhD
Resident Physician, Department of Plastic
Surgery, University of Pittsburgh Medical
Center, Pittsburgh, Pennsylvania

ANJALI C. RAGHURAM, MD
Resident Physician, Department of Plastic
Surgery, University of Pittsburgh Medical
Center, Pittsburgh, Pennsylvania

EVA ROY, MD
Resident Physician, Division of Plastic Surgery,
Massachusetts General Hospital, Harvard
Mass General Brigham Plastic Surgery;
Resident Physician, Clinical Fellow in Surgery,
Harvard Medical School, Boston,
Massachusetts

LUX SHAH, MD, MPH
Resident, UT Southwestern Department of
Surgery, University of Texas Southwestern
Medical Center, Dallas, Texas

GUY M. STOFMAN, MD, FACS
Co-Director Pitt Plastic Surgery Aesthetic
Center, Chief and Clinical Professor,
Department of Plastic Surgery, UPMC Mercy,
University of Pittsburgh Medical Center,
Pittsburgh, Pennsylvania

SAI R. VELAMURI, MD, FACS
Associate Professor, Department of Surgery,
College of Medicine, The University of
Tennessee Health Science Center, Memphis,
Tennessee

MOHAMED YASSIN, MD, PhD, MBA
Associate Professor of Medicine, Infectious
Diseases and Microbiology, University of
Pittsburgh School of Medicine and Public
Health, Medical Director, Infection Prevention
and Healthcare Epidemiology, UPMC Mercy,
Chief of Infectious Diseases UPMC Mercy,
Chair Quality Committee UPMC Mercy,
University of Pittsburgh Medical Center,
Pittsburgh, Pennsylvania

JENNY A. ZIEMBICKI, MD, FACS
Associate Professor, Director of UPMC Mercy
Burn Center, Department of Surgery, UPMC
Mercy, Pittsburgh, Pennsylvania

Contents

Burn care evolved slowly from primitive treatments depicted in cave drawings 3500 years ago to a vibrant medical specialty which has made remarkable progress over the past 200 years. This evolution involved all areas of burn care including superficial dressings, wound assessment, fluid resuscitation, infection control, pathophysiology, nutritional support, burn surgery, and inhalation injury. Major advances that contributed to current standards of care and improved outcomes are highlighted in this article. New innovations are making possible a future where severe burn injuries will require less morbid interventions for acute care and outcomes will restore patients more closely to their pre-injury condition.

Acute burn injury creates a complex and multifactorial local response which may have systemic sequelae such as hypovolemia, hypothermia, cardiovascular collapse, hypercoagulability, and multi-system organ failure. Understanding the underlying pathophysiology of burn shock, the initial burn triage and assessment, calculation of fluid requirements, and the means of tailoring ongoing interventions to optimize resuscitation are critical for overcoming the wide spectrum of derangements which this condition creates. As a result, this article discusses the various key points in order to garner a greater understanding of these nuances and the optimal pathway to take when tackling these challenging issues.

Sustaining an inhalation injury increases the risk of severe complications and mortality. Current evidential support to guide treatment of the injury or subsequent complications is lacking, as studies either exclude inhalation injury or design limit inferences that can be made. Conventional ventilator modes are most commonly used, but there is no consensus on optimal strategies. Settings should be customized to patient tolerance and response. Data for pharmacotherapy adjunctive treatments are limited.

Burn injuries affect patients of all ages, and timely surgical debridement and excision commence to protect dermal vascularity and integrity, improve healing, and minimize scarring. Several tools may be used for burn wound excision, which is performed either tangentially or down to muscular fascia. Once wounds are optimized from a tissue viability and healing standpoint, coverage may be obtained through grafts or secondary intention healing for more superficial injuries. A collaborative team of plastic and general surgeons, anesthesiologists, nutritionists, and therapists can provide improved patient care throughout the perioperative period, leading to improvements in overall patient morbidity and mortality.

Coverage of burn wounds is crucial to prevent sequalae including dehydration, wound infection, sepsis, shock, scarring, and contracture. To this end, numerous temporary and permanent options for coverage of burn wounds have been described. Temporary options for burn coverage include synthetic dressings, allografts, and xenografts. Permanent burn coverage can be achieved through skin substitutes, cultured epithelial autograft, ReCell, amnion, and autografting. Here, we aim to summarize the available options for burn coverage, as well as important considerations that must be made when choosing the best reconstructive option for a particular patient.

The leading cause of morbidity in burn patients is infection with pneumonia, urinary tract infection, cellulitis, and wound infection being the most common cause. High mortality is due to the immunocompromised status of patients and abundance of multidrug-resistant organisms in burn units. Despite the criteria set forth by American Association of Burn, the diagnosis and treatment of burn infections are not always straightforward. Topical antimicrobials, isolation, hygiene, and personal protective equipment are common preventive measures. Additionally medical and nutritional optimization of the patients is crucial to reverse the immunocompromised status triggered by burn injury.

Burn-related pain can contribute to decreased quality of life and long-term morbidity, limiting functional recovery. Burn-related pain should be assessed first by chronicity (acute or chronic), followed by type (nociceptive, neuropathic, nociplastic), to guide multimodal pharmacologic management in a stepwise algorithm approach. Combination therapies increase the efficacy and reduce toxicity by offering a multimodal approach that targets different receptors in the peripheral nervous system and central nervous system. When multimodal pharmacologic management is ineffective, etiologies of burn-related pain amenable to surgical interventions must be considered. It is important to know when to refer a patient to pain management.

Cold-induced injuries are a major challenge for burn surgeons, leading to significant sequelae for the patients including amputations, long-term disability, and death. Rapid assessment and diagnosis are essential for optimal outcomes. Various therapies have emerged to improve outcomes. Topical, oral, and intravenous agents have shown to minimize the impact of cold-induced injuries. Thrombolytics have shown the greatest promise in improving tissue perfusion outcomes in cold-induced injuries. This article provides an update on the evidence-based assessment and management of cold-induced injuries, as well as reviews outcomes and future directions of this challenging pathology.

Burns in the elderly are a significant cause of morbidity and mortality. Frailty is an important indicator of patient health and physiologic reserve. Comorbidities and typical age-related changes significantly impact the outcomes of elderly burn patients and decisions made during their burn care. It is essential to have early and thorough discussions about the goals of care and rehabilitation plans. Physiologic changes that occur from aging cause slower wound healing and may make operative treatment more challenging, although techniques such as autographing, skin substitutes, and flaps may all play a role in treating this patient population.

Large burns provoke profound pathophysiological changes. Survival rates of patients with large burns have improved significantly with the advancement of critical care and adaptation of early excision protocols. Nevertheless, care of large burn wounds remains challenging secondary to limited donor sites, prolonged time to wound closure, and immunosuppression. The development of skin substitutes and new grafting techniques decreased time to wound closure. Individually, these methods have limited success, but a combination of them may yield more successful outcomes. Early identification of patients with likely poor prognosis should prompt goals of care discussion and involvement of a palliative care team when possible.

CLINICS IN PLASTIC SURGERY

SERIES OF RELATED INTEREST

Facial Plastic Surgery Clinics
https://www.facialplastic.theclinics.com/
Otolaryngologic Clinics
https://www.oto.theclinics.com/
Advances in Cosmetic Surgery
www.advancesincosmeticsurgery.com/

Dedication

Acute and Reconstructive Burn Care: Part I

To my extraordinary mother, who gave me the gift of dreams and the ability to fulfill them. Your sacrifices and enduring love have been the heartbeat of my journey as a surgeon and have been the inspiration behind these pages. With gratitude,

Francesco M. Egro

To my parents, who believed in me before I did, and who provided me a foundation built on curiosity, kindness, and integrity.

C. Scott Hultman

Clin Plastic Surg 51 (2024) ix
https://doi.org/10.1016/j.cps.2023.12.002
0094-1298/24/© 2023 Published by Elsevier Inc.

Preface
Acute and Reconstructive Burn Care

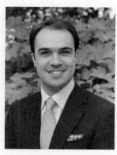
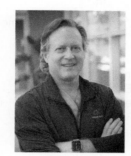

Francesco M. Egro, MD, MSc, MRCS   C. Scott Hultman, MD, MBA, FACS

Editors

Burn injuries pose one of the greatest challenges to health care professionals worldwide, requiring a multidisciplinary approach for optimal patient care. We are constantly reminded of the sheer resilience of the human spirit in the face of unimaginable pain and adversity experienced by these patients. It is with great passion and dedication that health care professionals strive to make a difference in the lives of those who have faced the inferno of acute burn injuries. This issue is dedicated to all the exceptional members of the burn team that deliver such incredible care with empathy, compassion, and unwavering commitment to our patients' well-being.

The field of burn surgery encompasses a wide range of knowledge and skills, from initial assessment and resuscitation to wound management, reconstructive procedures, and long-term rehabilitation. It is a field in constant evolution through research and innovation. This two-volume issue of *Clinics in Plastic Surgery* aims to serve as a comprehensive updated guide for burn surgeons and health care providers involved in the care of burn patients. Our goal in compiling this issue is to bring together a collection of expert insights and practical information that would not only address the fundamental principles of burn surgery but also provide valuable updates on emerging techniques and advancements in the field. Each article offers a comprehensive overview of the subject matter, supported by evidence-based approaches. Our aim is to provide readers with a clear understanding of the principles, techniques, and challenges involved in burn surgery, enabling them to deliver optimal care to burn patients and improve outcomes. We recognize that burn surgery is a dynamic and evolving field, with ongoing advancements in research and technology. Therefore, we have included articles that delve into the latest innovations and future directions in burn care, ensuring that readers stay abreast of the latest developments and are inspired to contribute to the progress of this field.

We hope that this issue serves as a valuable resource for burn surgeons, plastic surgeons, trauma surgeons, intensivists, nurses, therapists, and all health care professionals involved in the care of burn patients. It is our sincere hope that the knowledge shared within these pages will contribute to the advancement of burn surgery and, ultimately, lead to improved outcomes and quality of life for burn survivors.

Finally, we would like to extend our heartfelt gratitude to all the incredible contributors from all over

Clin Plastic Surg 51 (2024) xi–xii
https://doi.org/10.1016/j.cps.2023.10.001
0094-1298/24/© 2023 Published by Elsevier Inc.

the world, who have dedicated their time and expertise to make these issues possible. Their commitment to the field of burn surgery is commendable, and we are grateful for their contributions.

Francesco M. Egro, MD, MSc, MRCS
Associate Professor Department of Plastic
Surgery & Department of Surgery
Deputy Chief of Plastic Surgery UPMC Mercy
Associate Director of UPMC Mercy Burn Center
Director of Burn Reconstruction
Director of Medical Student Education
Associate Program Director Integrated &
Independent Residency
University of Pittsburgh Medical Center,
Pittsburgh, PA, USA

C. Scott Hultman, MD, MBA, FACS
WPP Plastic and Reconstructive Surgery
WakeMed Health and Hospitals
Raleigh, NC, USA

Campbell University
Buies Creek, NC, USA

Department of Plastic and Reconstructive Surgery
Johns Hopkins University
Baltimore, MD, USA

E-mail addresses:
francescoegro@gmail.com (F.M. Egro)
chultman@wakemed.org (C.S. Hultman)

Evolution of Burn Care
Past, Present, and Future

Martin R. Buta, MD, MBA[a,b,c], Matthias B. Donelan, MD[a,b,c],*

KEYWORDS

• Burns • Burn care • Thermal injury • Burn wound • Burn reconstruction • Skin substitutes • History

KEY POINTS

- Current burn care can only be understood and improved by knowing the past, critiquing the present, and having an open mind for the future.
- All areas of burn care and prevention have improved over the past 200 years. This progress has resulted in decreased mortality and improved quality of life for survivors.
- Hypertrophic and contracted scars are often the patient's most valuable reconstructive anatomy.
- Advances in lasers, skin substitutes, tissue engineering, and regenerative medicine are expanding treatment options.
- Most burn patients do not have access to state-of-the-art care. Preventable deaths and deformities occur world-wide because of this unfortunate fact.

INTRODUCTION

Burn injuries have been part of the human experience since *Homo sapiens* first walked the earth. The earliest recorded evidence of human burns and their treatment was found in cave paintings more than 3500 years old.[1] Today, burn injuries remain one of the leading causes of mortality and disability in the world. In 2019, there were more than 9.0 million burn cases severe enough to require medical attention. The World Health Organization has estimated there are approximately 180,000 deaths annually due to burns. Most burn injuries occur in low and middle-income countries, and almost two-thirds occur in the African and Southeast Asian regions. The global burden of burn trauma has remained persistently high, but survival rates and patient quality of life after burns have improved significantly over the past 150 years.[2] Unfortunately, because the majority of burns occur in disadvantaged countries, the improved treatments and outcomes that are now possible are often not available to patients in these countries.

Therapies for burn injuries described in the ancient literature were primarily superficial treatments. During the last several millennia, famous philosophers and physicians from many different cultures and civilizations have recommended myriad remedies and concoctions to treat burn wounds. All the recommended treatments may have provided a degree of patient comfort and cleanliness, but there is little to no evidence they improved outcomes or survival. The gradual onset of modern medicine with its more scientific approach to observed phenomena enabled progress to be made in the clinical care of burn injuries and the subsequent correction of the resulting deformities. The general acceptance of the germ theory of disease, heavily influenced by the seminal work of Louis Pasteur and later Robert Koch in the late 1800s, helped physicians begin to understand the role of the festering burn wound itself as the origin of infection and the source of the sepsis that led to patient death.[3,4]

Advances in surgery were made possible by the discovery of anesthesia during the nineteenth

[a] Plastic, Reconstructive, and Laser Surgery, Shriners Hospitals for Children, Boston, MA, USA; [b] Division of Plastic and Reconstructive Surgery, Massachusetts General Hospital, Boston, MA; [c] Harvard Medical School, Boston, MA, USA
* Corresponding author. Plastic, Reconstructive, and Laser Surgery, Shriners Hospitals for Children, 51 Blossom Street, Boston, MA 02114.
E-mail address: mdonelan@mgh.harvard.edu

Clin Plastic Surg 51 (2024) 191–204
https://doi.org/10.1016/j.cps.2023.10.002
0094-1298/24/© 2023 Elsevier Inc. All rights reserved.

century. The earliest evidence of plastic surgery goes back over 2000 years to India and the famous nasal reconstructions described by Sushruta (c. mid-1st millennium BC), but the dawn of modern plastic surgery can be traced back to local tissue rearrangements in the 1800s to correct burn contractures.[5] The contractures frequently resulted from burn wounds that could only heal by contraction and epithelialization.[6] Anesthesia enabled burn survivors to have disabling scar contractures improved by using their own local scar tissue as the reconstructive material. This was the beginning of a continuous era of progress in local scar tissue rehabilitation that persists today and incorporates further advances in surgical techniques and new technologies.

Understanding the evolution of burn care from its earliest beginnings to the present day requires knowledge of the history of science and medicine over that same period. It was impossible in the 1600s to understand why some patients lived and some patients died from burn wounds that looked very much the same. The physicians and practitioners who worked on solving those mysteries were heroes. Pursuing progress in closed-minded societies, ruled by despots, required courage and determination. Galileo, in 1632, did not believe that the sun revolved around the earth and published the reasons why. His reward was excommunication and house arrest for the remainder of his life.

The evolution of burn care can only be understood and appreciated by knowing its history and context.

TOPICAL TREATMENTS, THE BASIS OF EARLY BURN CARE

Burn injuries are primarily superficial and so it is not surprising that for the first 2000 years of recorded medical history, the management of burns focused primarily on topical treatments. Two medical texts from Ancient Egypt are among the earliest documents on burn wound therapy. The Edwin Smith Papyrus, written in 1600 BC, noted the use of therapeutic ointment made from resin and honey. The even more comprehensive Ebers Papyrus, written in 1550 BC, described a topical concoction made from cattle dung, bees wax, ram's horn, and barley porridge soaked in resin for treating burn wounds.[7–9]

Various civilizations around the globe developed assorted topical therapies. In 600 BC, the Chinese used tea leaf extracts for burn injuries. The ancient Greeks also made notable contributions. In 200 B.C., the famous philosopher and physician Hippocrates described wound dressings made with rendered pig fat and resin that were alternated with vinegar soaks augmented with tanning solutions derived from oak bark. Celsus, another Greek philosopher who lived in the 1st century AD, recommended the application of a lotion made from wine and myrrh to burn wounds, possibly for their bacteriostatic properties.[7] Galen (130–210 CE) mentioned a burn therapy based on vinegar and exposure of the burn wound to air. The Arabian physician Rhases (865–925 CE), also known as Abu Bakr Muhammad Ibn Zakariya Al Razi, was the first to mention first aid for burns using cold water to provide pain relief.[7] Ambroise Paré (1510–1590), a French barber surgeon who served in that role for several kings, described using onions and early wound excision for treating burns.[10,11] In his book, De Combustionibus, the German physician Wilhelm Fabricius Hildanus (1560–1634), considered the father of surgery in Germany, explained burn pathophysiology and his approach to treating burn contractures.[7,12] In 1797, Edward Kentish, a British surgeon, detailed in an essay focused on burn injuries in mine workers, how pressure dressings could be used to alleviate burn pain.[13]

There is no evidence that any of the topical dressings and various treatments described during this long period had any positive effect on survival from the burn injury, probably because they had little to no effect on bacterial contamination and infections which were not understood.

BURN DEPTH CLASSIFICATION

For several millennia, there was no consistent and widely used nomenclature for characterizing burn wounds. A milestone was achieved in 1634 when Wilhelm Hildanus described the association of tissue injury and the duration of heat exposure. His description was the first recorded instance of burn depth classification. He proposed 3 stages: the first involved erythema and blisters filled with clear fluid, the second involved erythema and blisters filled with yellow fluid, and the third was characterized by painless firm, dry skin colored black or blue and absent of any blistering.[7,12] Several decades later, in 1681, Van Alberding similarly utilized a 3-stage classification for burn depth. He described a first stage of light burns with blistering, a second stage of skin contraction, and a third stage of ulceration and crusting with skin separation.[14]

The introduction of the term "degrees" in classifying burns came in the 18th century, when the German surgeons Heister (1724) and Richter (1788) described four degrees for burn injuries: the first degree entailed small blisters accompanied by heat and pain; the second degree involved large blisters and significant pain; the third degree involved crust formation overlying damaged skin and the supportive soft tissues; and the fourth degree entailed soft tissue damage extending to the bone.[14] A French surgeon, Alexis Boyer, proposed a three-degree system in 1814.[15] In 1839, another French surgeon, Guillaume Dupuytren, published a study on 50 burn patients in which he proposed a classification for burn depth defined by six degrees, but his system lost favor to simpler classifications.[16] Today, the four-degree classification adopted during the 20th century is being countered by a system that describes burns by depth: superficial, superficial partial thickness, deep partial thickness, and full thickness. Classifying the depth of burn wounds by observation and physical examination is a challenging task. The heterogenous nature of most wounds and the subjectivity in making an assessment can cause significant inter-observer variability, particularly when distinguishing between deep second-degree and third-degree.

Laser doppler imaging (LDI) was a great leap forward in this area. LDI objectively and accurately assesses microcirculation within dermal tissue and has been approved for clinical evaluation of burn depth by regulatory bodies, including the Food and Drug Administration (FDA). In 1993, Niazi and colleagues found a high correlation of clinical, histologic, and LDI measurements of wound depth. This was the first study to report using LDI to objectively and accurately measure burn depth.[17] There is persisting skepticism about LDI and a reluctance to utilize it at many burn centers. Claes and colleagues stated, in their 2021 paper, *The LDI Enigma, Part I: So much proof, so little use*: "Barriers for the implementation of LDI are: (1) cost of purchasing and using an LDI combined with healthcare systems that inadequately reimburse conservative management; (2) lack of awareness of, or ongoing skepticism toward the scientific evidence supporting LDI use; and (3) organizational constraints combined with logistical limitations."[18,19] Burn units that have adopted LDI technology have reported a decreased incidence of acute burn excision and grafting.[20] This is important progress. Improved methods of burn scar rehabilitation are available today and will likely be further improved in the future. It may be harmful to patients to perform acute excision and grafting for non-life-threatening burns.[21] Multiple other technologies have also been introduced over the past 30 years to provide objective and accurate burn depth evaluations. These new technologies include near infrared spectroscopy, laser speckled imaging, and spatial frequency domain imaging.[14,17,18,22–25]

BURN WOUND SURFACE AREA

The recognition of an association between a burn wound's dimensions and mortality is a relatively recent development in the burn care story. In 1876, C. Smart published a study on 12 individuals injured from a gunpowder explosion on a ship, noting the connection of wound depth and size, among other measures, to burn severity.[26] In 1884, Schjerning proposed that death would result if two-thirds of the body was burned and death was expected if half of the body was burned.[27]

In 1879, Meeh described an approach to measure body surface area (BSA) using paper. This technique proved impractical but established the idea of BSA.[28] Weidenfeld refined the approach after realizing different parts of the body, such as the head or extremities, contributed a constant fraction to total BSA. Weidenfeld's technique permitted a more objective assessment of burn size, which he linked to mortality along with burn depth, age, and general health.[29]

In the late 1800s and early 1900s, Berkow advanced the development of BSA by measuring the surface area of different body parts and relating them to total body surface area (TBSA). Berkow's work leveraged the calculations by D. Du Bois and E.F. Du Bois in which TBSA was a function of height and weight.[30] In 1944, Lund and Browder created a chart that is widely used today in trauma and burn centers to assess the surface area for a burn. The Lund and Browder chart includes 12 regions of the body that each contributes a fraction of TBSA along with an age correction factor for children.[14,31] In 1951, A.B. Wallace, a Scottish plastic surgeon, influenced by the work of Berkow, and later Pulaski and Tennison, published a paper describing the "Rule of Nines" as a practical and relatively rapid method to approximate the total body surface area affected by a burn.[32] The Rule of Nines is still commonly used today although its shortcomings are well known, especially in obese and pediatric burn patients. These limitations have motivated many studies assessing 3D imaging devices and software designed to calculate TBSA.[33–35]

FLUID RESUSCITATION

The significance of fluid losses and electrolyte imbalances resulting from burn injuries was first appreciated by F.P. Underhill at Yale while studying blister fluid in 20 patients burned in the 1921 Rialto Theater fire. He discovered that the fluid was similar in composition to that of plasma and suggested early mortality from burns was a consequence not of toxins but of fluid losses due to increased capillary permeability. In addition, he proposed using the blood hemoglobin percentage as an indicator of resuscitative needs.[36] Over the next 2 decades, building on Underhill's concept of thermal injury-induced intravascular fluid deficits and informed by new tools to assess TBSA, such as the Lund and Browder chart and Rule of Nines, various approaches to fluid replacement were developed. Casualties involving burns during World War II served as a significant impetus to improve resuscitation protocols and fluids.

From their studies of burn patients injured in Boston's Coconut Grove Nightclub fire in 1942, Cope and Moore established the relationship between the percent body surface area burned and the fluid volume needed for resuscitation. In 1947, they proposed a revision of the National Research Council resuscitation formula called the Surface Area Formula.[37,38] Moore later described the Burn Budget Formula to calculate the volume of fluid to be administered for a given surface area burned, recognizing that fluid losses in burn patients were due not only to evaporative water loss and fluids absorbed by bed sheets, but by "third space" losses.[39]

After World War II, various resuscitation formulas were devised, incorporating different volumes per weight per TBSA and combinations of crystalloid and colloid. In 1952, Evans and colleagues described the Evans formula, which added body weight to surface area burned for calculating resuscitative volumes.[40] Baxter and Shires developed what is now the most widely used formula, the Parkland formula, which recommends 4 mL of lactated Ringer's solution per kg/% TBSA burned given during the first 24 hours after burn injury, with half of the fluid administered in the first 8 hours.[41]

INFECTION CONTROL

The theory of spontaneous generation, or life arising from nonliving matter, was eventually debunked by Pasteur's work, giving way to the modern germ theory of disease. Improved survival came with the development of topical and systemic antimicrobial agents that could help control bacterial proliferation in the festering burn wounds, and the bacteremia that led to organ failure and death. The beginning of progress in this area was the use of sodium hypochlorite, a topical antimicrobial discovered in the 18th century and commonly used as a disinfectant in the 19th century. Unfortunately, the use of this agent was limited by skin irritation due to the free alkali or chlorine it contained.[42] In 1915, Henry D. Dakin refined the ingredients of the solution to eliminate irritating contaminants. Dakin worked with French surgeon and Nobel Prize winner Alexis Carrel to develop a protocol for treating wounds and burns with mechanical cleansing, surgical debridement, and topical application of sodium hypochlorite solution. The protocol became integral to clinical care for soldiers injured in World War I who were frequently dying from wound infections. Dakin's solution was very effective and popular, as was evidenced by numerous military hospitals opening Carrel-Dakin Wards during World War I. The effectiveness of Dakin's solution is compromised by its rapid inactivation, limited wound penetration, and local toxicity.[43–45]

The broad-spectrum antimicrobial agent, mafenide acetate (Sulfamylon), was first used by microbiologist Robert Lindberg and surgeon John Moncrief to treat burn wounds. It was able to quickly penetrate third-degree burn eschar and effectively reduce bacterial burden. Unfortunately, it could potentially result in systemic acidosis and pulmonary edema, impeding its adoption except in cases involving invasive wound infection.[46,47] The introduction of silver-based topical therapies was a breakthrough in burn treatment. Silver sulfadiazine cream (Silvadene), developed by Charles Fox in the 1960s, became central to burn care given its ability to reduce sepsis and mortality associated with burn wounds.[47,48] In their landmark study in 1965, Moyer and Monafo reported on the antimicrobial efficacy of 0.5% silver nitrate soaks in large burn wounds. Since then, silver nitrate soaks have been widely adopted by burn centers.[49]

In 1928, Scottish scientist Sir Alexander Fleming discovered penicillin's antimicrobial properties. Remarkably, it was only after the development of large-scale manufacturing of the drug during World War II that its use became widespread. With the emergence of penicillin-resistant bacteria able to cleave the penicillin's beta-lactam ring, newer penicillinase-resistant penicillins were required and developed, such as methicillin in the 1950s and cloxacillin in the 1960s.

In addition to topical and systemic antibiotics, many other approaches have been used to mitigate against infection and prevent cross contamination from burn patients including patient isolation, frequent handwashing, early burn wound excision, burn unit design, and bacterial control nursing units (BCNUs), first described by John F. Burke and colleagues in 1977.[14,50] In spite of these developments, today sepsis remains a fundamental concern, as it is the leading cause of mortality in burn patients, playing a role in 75% to 85% of all burn patient deaths.[51]

BURN SURGERY

Ambroise Paré first wrote about acute burn wound excision in the 1500s. Wilhelm Hildanus also recommended excision in the 1600s. Early excision, however, fell into disfavor due to high infection rates and blood loss.[12,14] There was a basic understanding that necrotic tissue contributed to the patient's systemic illness but fear of patient intraoperative death from hemorrhage, and the inability to close open wounds, prevented early excision. This left burn patients, especially those with major injuries, to heal their wounds by bacterial eschar separation and multiple small debridements of necrotic tissue. When skin grafting became available in the 1800s the open, granulating, wounds could be closed with grafts. The eschar separation process required a prolonged clinical course and resulted in malnutrition, contractures, and severe disabilities.[14]

Many surgeons made important contributions to skin grafting techniques in the 1800s. Christian Bunger, a German surgeon, is considered by many to have carried out the first skin graft in Europe in 1823. Inspired by the ancient Indian method in which thick skin from the buttock was grafted onto a nasal defect, Bunger reconstructed a nasal wound using full-thickness skin from the thigh.[52,53] Jonathan Mason Warren, an American surgeon at Massachusetts General Hospital, reported in 1840 using full-thickness skin to repair a nasal defect.[52,54] In 1869, the Swiss surgeon Jacques-Louis Reverdin described the use of "epidermal grafting" on granulating wounds by harvesting the grafts from pinched skin.[52,55] In 1870, British surgeon George Pollock reported the first successful case of using skin grafts on a burn wound.[52] In 1872, the French Surgeon Louis Ollier published his work using strips of split-thickness skin grafts that were larger than those used by Reverdin and Pollock.[56] In 1875, the Scottish ophthalmologist J.R. Wolfe described in the British Medical Journal the technique of full-thickness skin grafting for ophthalmic defects like entropion.[52,55] Building on the studies by Ollier, Karl Thiersch, a German surgeon, developed a technique for split-thickness skin grafts that was widely adopted and remained popular until the 1940s.[52,55,56]

Skin grafting in the 1800s resulted in grafts of variable thickness because they were harvested freehand using a knife with a long blade and attached handle. Early examples included the Blair knife, Catlin knife, and Ferris-Smith knife.[57] Multiple innovations paved the way to today's grafting instruments and techniques which harvest predictable grafts of uniform thickness. Thomas Humby, in the early 1930s, improved the Blair knife

by adding a roller in front of the blade and a new handle. In 1955, Fenton Braithwaite modified one of Humby's designs to include a replaceable blade. In 1960, John Watson made the roller guard adjustable to set the graft thickness which then could be locked in place (**Fig. 1**). Dicran Goulian introduced a knife system that included a fixed handle to a Weck blade and interchangeable spacers to adjust graft thickness. Otto Lanz, a Swiss surgeon, is credited with first introducing meshed skin grafts in 1907, using the Hautschlitzapparat, a device he invented that was covered with small, parallel knives.[52,55] E.C. Padgett invented the adjustable drum dermatome in the late 1930s. His device was improved by John Davies Reese into the Padgett-Hood dermatome in the 1940s to allow greater precision and reliability in obtaining a given graft thickness. The first mechanical dermatome was electric powered and developed in the late 1940s by Harry M. Brown. In 1958, C.P. Meek achieved a 9-fold expansion of harvested skin using the Meek-Wall dermatome, which proved to be difficult to use. Current enhanced versions of the Meek technique have potential for improvement in both functional and esthetic skin graft outcomes because of the small size of the individual grafts. Probably the most revolutionary grafting technology came in 1964, when J.C Tanner and colleagues introduced the skin graft meshing device, which created a 3:1 expansion of donor skin and has become the most commonly used technique for acute burn grafting.[14,52,55,57,58]

During World War II when military hospitals saw a dramatic rise in the number of burn patients, physicians began to report improved mortality rates after early excision of burn eschar followed by grafting.[59] In the 1950s, Douglas Jackson and colleagues at Birmingham Accident Hospital demonstrated that immediate excision and grafting (20%–30% TBSA) was safe to carry out when shock was well controlled.[60] Jackson's results were impressive but surgeons remained resistant because of continued fear of infection and blood loss. Large burns were typically addressed with delayed serial excision.

Zora Janzekovic published a paper in 1970 which created a new concept for early excision

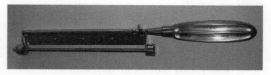

Fig. 1. Watson knife. (*From* Jeffery SL. Device related tangential excision in burns. Injury. 2007 Dec;38 Suppl 5:S35–8. PMID: 18061188.)

and grafting (**Fig. 2**). She reported her experience in 2,615 patients using early tangential excision to remove eschar from small, deep second-degree burns down to bleeding tissues with immediate autografting 3 to 5 days after injury.[61] Evidence supporting early tangential excision accumulated rapidly after her report. W. Monafo advocated in 1974 for using the technique in larger burns. John F. Burke and colleagues demonstrated markedly improved survival rates in children with burns greater than 80% TBSA.[62,63] In 1988, Ronald G. Tompkins and colleagues reported an extraordinary decrease in mortality in children with severe burns who were treated with early excision and grafting.[64] David Herndon and colleagues reported in 1989 that lower mortality rates were achieved in patients treated with early excision compared to conservative management.[65]

Early surgical debridement has now become an integral part of acute burn care. Unfortunately, the accurate identification and excision of necrotic tissue while still preserving healthy tissue in mixed-depth wounds is a challenge for even the most experienced surgeons.[66] The shortcomings of excisional debridement include suboptimal tissue

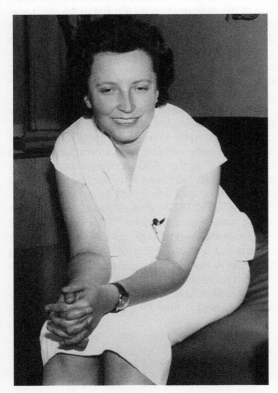

Fig. 2. The young Slovenian physician Zora Janzekovic. (*From* Janzekovic Z. Once upon a time how west discovered east. J Plast Reconstr Aesthet Surg. 2008;61(3):240–4. PMID: 18243082; with permission.)

preservation, major blood loss, iatrogenic injury to viable tissues, and impaired function and cosmesis.[67] Because of these surgical limitations, enzymatic debridement has been extensively investigated. Neutral proteases made from *Bacillus subtilis* (sutilains) were first described in 1969 and the sutilain product Travase gained some traction in the 1970s and 1980s.[68,69] Enzymes derived from plant extracts were first used for eschar removal in the 1940s. Bromelain-based enzymatic debridement (BBED), using an agent derived from pineapples, has gained popularity in burn centers in Europe in the last decade. Numerous studies have reported on the safety and efficacy of BBED in removing necrotic eschar from deep part-thickness and full-thickness burn wounds after a single application.[68,70]

Early tangential excision and grafting led to a paradigm shift in burn care with significant increases in survival rates. Many other important developments also increased survival. In the 1940 to 50s, glycerol-based cryopreservation and long-term storage of human skin was developed to facilitate wound closure in patients with burns greater than 50% TBSA in which available donor sites were inadequate.[71] In 1971, Bondoc and Burke advanced the field of cryopreservation, reporting on their techniques for the long-term storage of large quantities of frozen human skin.[71]

The limitations imposed by autografts and allografts served as an impetus to develop skin substitutes. The research of Yannas and Burke in the 1970s lead to the first artificial skin, Integra®, consisting of a silastic epidermis and a collagen-chondroitin dermis.[72] Since its FDA approval in 1996 and widespread adoption, Integra® has been followed by multiple other skin substitutes on the market.[73]

The treatment of burn scars has had a remarkable evolution over the past 200 years. Before general anesthesia was discovered in 1846, and local anesthesia in 1884, patients with burn scars and contractures had limited treatment options. They were largely forced to accept their appearance and disabilities.[74] In 1829, prior to anesthesia, J.C. Fricke released an upper eyelid contracture and closed the resulting defect with a local transposition flap from the forehead (**Fig. 3**). In 1842, again prior to anesthesia, Thomas Mutter released a severe anterior neck contracture and closed the open wound with a transposition flap from the shoulder carried out under hypnosis (**Fig 4**).[75,76] The donor sites for Fricke's and Mutter's patients were left open to heal by contraction and epithelialization. After anesthesia became available, local tissue rearrangement operations were frequently performed to ameliorate burn scar contractures

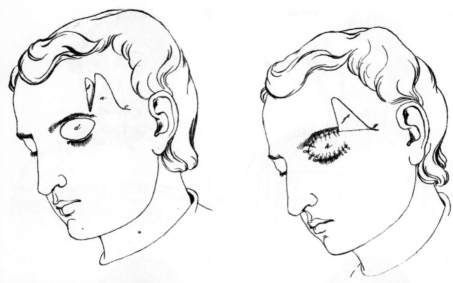

Fig. 3. Fricke's flap for periorbital reconstruction. (*A*) Burn scar contracture of the neck. (*B*) Contracture release. (*C*) Inset of mastoid-occiput-based shoulder flap. (*D*) 12 months postop with no contracture evident in the flap. Fricke's flap for periorbital reconstruction. (From Fricke JCG. Die Bildung neuer Augenlider (Blepharoplastik) nach Zerstörungen und dadurch hervorgebrachten Auswärtswendung derselben. Hamburg; Perthes & Besser. 1829.)

and improve appearance. Horner was reportedly the first to use a Z-plasty in 1837 to address a lower eyelid ectropion, followed by Denonvilliers in 1854. Anesthesia made possible more complex innovations in surgical techniques, such as the double transposition Z-plasty described by Berger in 1904. McCurdy was the first to use the term "Z-plastic operations" in 1913, which eventually became part of the plastic surgery lexicon as a "Z-plasty" (**Fig 5**).[75] Berger emphasized that with burn scar contractures, "the prime object is to preserve tissue. In no instance should any portion of the cicatricial band be removed."[75] J.S. Davis, in 1931, reiterated this point, stating "As we use the z-type incision the scar is not removed but the contraction is relieved by the transposition of flaps which are usually composed of scar or scar infiltrated tissue…"[77]

Despite these prescient observations about preserving burn scar tissue, surgeons during the 20th century used new anatomic knowledge and new techniques like microsurgery to excise scars and replace them with uninjured skin from other areas of patients' bodies. The pursuit of a scarless burn reconstruction was inspired by Sir Harold Gillies, the father of modern plastic surgery. He reported a World War I British army soldier whose facial burn scars were excised and replaced with a tubed pedicle flap of abdominal skin transferred by attaching it to his wrist.[78] This was a brilliant surgical innovation and was based on the premise that scar excision and closure with an unscarred

skin flap would give a better result than rehabilitating scarred skin or replacing it with skin grafts.[75] Many surgeons embraced Gillies' concept and reported impressive outcomes using many different flap techniques to close the defects after excision. Advances in surgical anatomy and operative skills enabled progressively larger scar excisions and flap closures that culminated in facial transplantation.[79] Scar removal per se became a goal of burn reconstruction surgery. Scar excision and graft closure of the resulting defects was also frequently used as better grafting techniques and devices became available. Experience unfortunately demonstrated that excision and closure surgery can result in changes that make patients look deformed in different ways rather than restored more closely to their pre-injury condition. Donor sites are also iatrogenic injuries which have morbidity and complications of their own.

20th-century burn reconstruction was dominated by scar excision and flap closure following Gillies' influence. Albert Einstein proposed his theory of relativity in 1905 and 1915, which led to the first therapeutic laser (ruby) in 1960.[80] T. Alster, a dermatologist, made a pivotal contribution to burn care in 1994 when she reported that the pulsed-dye laser could be used to treat hypertrophic, erythematous, painful, and pruritic scars.[81] Using the concepts of selective photothermolysis and fractional thermolysis, laser scar rehabilitation provides a revolutionary alternative to surgically removing scars.[82,83] Instead of excising scars,

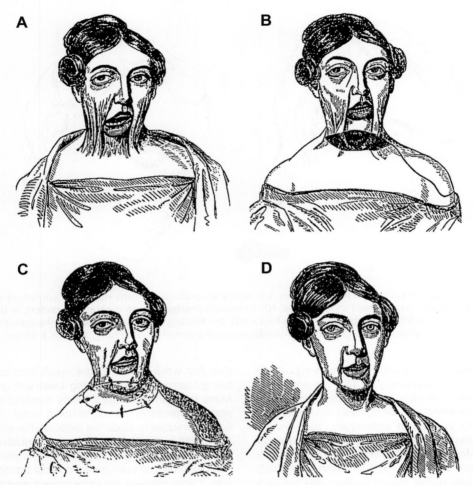

Fig. 4. Mutter's reconstruction. (*A*) Burn scar contracture of the neck. (*B*) Contracture release. (*C*) Inset of mastoid-occiput-based shoulder flap. (*D*) 12 months postop with no contracture evident in the flap. (*From* Mutter TD. Cases of deformities from burns, relieved by operation. Am J Med Sci 1842;4:66–90.)

lasers stimulate the healing properties of a patient's tissue, and induce it to remodel and regenerate. When used in conjunction with simple, classic plastic surgery, such as Z-plasties and local flaps to decrease tension and reorient scars, scars can blend so well into the adjacent tissue that excisional surgery is rarely indicated. The first paper recommending this approach as an alternative to burn scar excision was published in 2008.[84] Patients and families are grateful to have this option. The rehabilitation of the injured normal skin in its normal location can give results superior to flaps from distant sites that do not match the adjacent skin (**Box 1**). Laser-assisted drug delivery, following treatment with fractional ablative CO2 lasers, can also rehabilitate hypertrophic and contracted scars. All of these less morbid treatments improve scar elasticity and morphology and help to camouflage the scarred areas.[85–89]

Laser devices have now been used for over 30 years to provide state-of-the-art care to patients who have sustained burn injuries. There is extensive evidence in the literature, both clinical and experimental, that strongly supports the efficacy of laser therapy for the management and rehabilitation of burns and burn scars. Despite this evidence, laser therapy for burn care has not been universally accepted as standard of care.[84,89] Fifty years ago, virtually every burn scar operation began by excising the offending scar tissue. Today, that strategy is antiquated and should be avoided whenever possible. There is nothing like original equipment.

HYPERMETABOLISM AND NUTRITIONAL SUPPORT

John Hunter, the first academic surgeon, provided one of the first detailed descriptions of inflammation

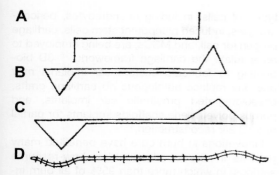

Fig. 5. To elongate a scar, McCurdy published in 1898 a zig-zag incision that later became known as a Z-plasty. (*From* McCurdy SL. Manual of Orthopedic Surgery. 1st ed. Pittsburgh; Nicholson Press. 1898.)

and the catabolic response to injury in a treatise published in 1794.[90] In the 1940s, another Scottish physician, D.P. Cuthbertson, made seminal contributions to our understanding of the "ebb and flow" metabolic response to injury, describing the hypometabolic state that occurs during the acute or shock phase and the subsequent hypermetabolic state during the chronic response phase.[91–93] In 1974, D. Wilmore and colleagues identified the primary role of catecholamines in the hypermetabolic response and in 1984, P.Q. Bessey found that cortisol and glucagon were also integral to the stress response.[94,95]

At the beginning of the 1900s, practitioners began to recognize the increased caloric needs of burn patients. P.A. Shaffer and W. Coleman encouraged high caloric intake after burn injury in 1909, but it wasn't until the 1970s that a comprehensive understanding emerged that adequate nutrition is essential to counter the hypermetabolic response.[96,97] In a retrospective study published in 1974, P.W. Curreri and colleagues determined the caloric intake needed for adult burn patients

---

Box 1
Advantages of Native Scar Tissue

A burn patient's most valuable reconstructive anatomy is often their own hypertrophic and contracted scars:

- It is autologous tissue.
- It is already in the right location.
- It is the closest match.
- Revising it requires no new donor sites.
- Revising it involves simple surgery.
- Revising it is minimally morbid.
- Revising it burns no bridges.

---

to maintain body weight for a given period of time.[98] In 1989, D.N. Herndon and colleagues reported a significantly higher mortality rate when patients with large burns were given intravenous supplementation of enteral calories versus enteral calories alone, thus he advocated intravenous supplemental nutrition only in patients whose enteral function has failed.[99]

In recent decades, various pharmacologic and hormonal interventions that reduce the hypermetabolic response and enhance nutritional support have been identified. β-adrenergic blockade has been shown to improve the metabolic response in pediatric burn patients.[100] By reducing proteolysis or stimulating protein synthesis, growth hormone, insulin-like growth factor 1, low dose insulin, metformin, and the testosterone analog oxandrolone have also demonstrated enhanced nutritional support.[101–106]

INHALATION INJURY

In the 1950s and 1960s, significant advances were made in understanding and treating burn shock, sepsis, kidney dysfunction, and burn wounds. Greater attention was focused on inhalation injury as patients increasingly survived their acute burn injuries. Inhalation injury was found to reflect 2 etiologies: a noninflammatory process caused by carbon monoxide poisoning and an inflammatory process that results from direct contact of the offending agent (eg, hot air, scalding liquid, and toxic biproducts from incomplete combustion such as aldehydes and ketones).[38] Studies by Foley and colleagues and Moylan and colleagues provided insights into sequelae that can develop in the first 24 hours after injury, such as upper airway obstruction and edema, and those that can develop after the initial 24-hour period, such pulmonary edema, tracheobronchitis, pneumonia, and airway plugs leading to occlusion.[1,107,108]

Inhalation injury, often presenting with nonspecific clinical signs and leading to pneumonia within a week of burn injury, motivated efforts to improve diagnostic techniques. Fiberoptic bronchoscopy, investigated by the US Army Burn Center, proved beneficial not only for pulmonary lavage but demonstrated an 86% accuracy in identifying inhalation injury. The accuracy improved to 93% with the addition of the xenon-133 ventilation-perfusion lung scan in burn patients with a negative bronchoscopy but suspected of smoke exposure.[109–111] Later studies by Sharani, Pruitt, and Mason reported that inhalation injury increased mortality up to 20% more than predicted based on a burn patient's age and burn size. The presence of pneumonia worsened mortality even more, up to

60% above the rate predicted by patient age and burn size.[112]

The treatment of inhalation injury has seen great progress over last 50 years, with successful therapeutic strategies focused on restoring and maintaining airway patency. High frequency intermittent positive-flow pressure ventilation was shown to facilitate the clearance of pulmonary secretions, minimize barotrauma, reduce the incidence of pneumonia, and improve survival.[113] Other therapeutic advances include various aerosolized bronchodilators; aerosolized heparin, which dissolves hemorrhagic casts that can obstruct airways, and N-acetyl-L-cysteine, which reduces inflammation caused by oxygen radicals and facilitates mucous clearance.[38] Future treatments to mitigate the secondary effects of inhalation injury will likely involve innovative drugs targeting mediators of the acute inflammatory response.

FUTURE DIRECTIONS

Future innovations in tissue engineering and regenerative medicine are necessary to continue the rapid progress achieved in burn care during the last century. Extensive research is currently focused on developing a skin substitute that will obviate the need for autologous skin grafts for all but the most extensive and deep burns.[114] Mixed second-degree burns that develop focal areas of scarring can now be rehabilitated in ways that were inconceivable 40 years ago. It is often easier to improve hypertrophic scarring than to improve areas that were acutely excised and grafted. Early excision and split-thickness skin grafts for non-life-threatening burns can lead to significant donor-site morbidity. There are very few studies in the literature that have assessed the incidence of this iatrogenic morbidity. A systematic review (2009–2019) noted only 1 long-term study that assessed permanent split-thickness donor site deformities. In that study, an 8-year follow-up revealed a 28% incidence of hypertrophic scarring.[21] This high rate and the preponderance of split-thickness skin grafts for non-life-threatening wounds warrant additional investigation and great care when treating small, superficial burns. Such patients may have better long-term outcomes without early excision for small burn injuries.

There are published studies exploring the application of allograft and autograft mesenchymal stem cells (MSCs) to wound healing, but the majority involving animals and human studies are lacking.[115]

For complex facial burns involving cartilaginous structures such as the ear and nose, different types of cells, including chondrocytes, pericondrocytes, induced pluripotent stem cells, cartilage progenitor cell, and MSCs, are being employed to recapitulate the cartilage framework.[116] 3D bioprinting to fabricate custom ear implants may one day replace autologous rib cartilage grafts, osseointegrated prosthetic ear implants, and porous polyethylene scaffolds implants for partial or total ear reconstruction.[117]

Innovations in burn care have benefited many patients in developed countries. Low-resource settings, in which more than 95% of all burn injuries occur, have yet to see many of these gains.[118,119] It is incumbent upon the burn care specialty to disseminate knowledge, devise practical and affordable advances to make burn care better, and to minimize further iatrogenic deformities as we strive to save lives and return patients as much as possible to their pre-injury condition.[118]

SUMMARY

Rudimentary observations, topical treatments, and procedures dominated burn care for millennia. The wide adoption of the scientific method and the acceptance of the germ theory of disease altered this trajectory, resulting in today's standard of care. Open-minded practitioners familiar with burn care's evolution, as well as its current challenges, are well-positioned to improve mortality rates and the quality of life of burn survivors.

CLINICS CARE POINTS

- Burn depth diagnosis remains highly subjective, particularly in distinguishing between superficial and deep second degree, the essential diagnosis. Laser doppler imaging (LDI) has been demonstrated to be accurate and results in a decreased incidence of acute burn excision and grafting.

- Rehabilitation of scarred normal skin in its normal location can give results superior to flaps and grafts which do not match adjacent skin. Rehabilitating scars with local plastic surgery, lasers, and topical treatments instead of excising them decreases morbidity and leads to patient satisfaction.

- Donor site morbidity from grafts and flaps used to reconstruct burn deformities is an iatrogenic injury and should be minimized whenever possible.

DISCLOSURE

The authors report no conflicts of interest or financial disclosures.

REFERENCES

1. Branski LK, Herndon DN, Barrow RE. A brief history of acute burn care management. In: Herndon DN, editor. Total burn care. 5th edition. Edinburgh: Saunders; 2018. p. 1–7.
2. Gerstl JVE, Ehsan AN, Lassaren P, et al. The global macroeconomic burden of burn injuries. Plast Reconstr Surg 2023.
3. Walker L, Levine H, Jucker M. Koch's postulates and infectious proteins. Acta Neuropathol 2006; 112(1):1–4.
4. Opal SM. The evolution of the understanding of sepsis, infection, and the host response: a brief history. Crit Care Clin 2009;25(4):637–63.
5. Puthumana PP. Through the mists of time: sushrutha, an enigma revisited. Indian J Plast Surg 2009;42(2):219–23.
6. Eger EI, Saidman LJ, Westhorpe R. The wondrous story of anesthesia, 944. New York: Springer; 2014. p. xviii.
7. Majno G. The healing hand: man and wound in the ancient world. Cambridge: Harvard University Press; 1975.
8. Stiefel M, Shaner A, Schaefer SD. The Edwin Smith Papyrus: the birth of analytical thinking in medicine and otolaryngology. Laryngoscope 2006;116(2): 182–8.
9. Bryan CP. The Papyrus Ebers. London: Geoffrey Bles; 1930.
10. Shen JT, Weinstein M, Beekley A, et al. Ambroise Pare (1510 to 1590): a surgeon centuries ahead of his time. Am Surg 2014;80(6):536–8.
11. Donaldson IM. Ambroise Pare's accounts of new methods for treating gunshot wounds and burns. J R Soc Med 2015;108(11):457–61.
12. Jones E. The life and works of guilhelmus Fabricius Hildanus. Med Hist 1960;4(2):112–134 contd.
13. Kentish E. An essay on burns : principally upon those which happpen to workmen in mines. G.G. and J. Robinson; 1797.
14. Lee KC, Joory K, Moiemen NS. History of burns: the past, present and the future. Burns Trauma 2014;2(4):169–80.
15. Boyer A. Traits of surgical diseases and operations of their choosing. Paris, Migneret: TI; 1814.
16. Dupuytren G, Brierre de Boismont AJF, Paillard ALM. Oral lessons of clinical surgery, faites à l'Hôtel-Dieu de Paris. Baillière Paris. 1839.
17. Niazi ZB, Essex TJ, Papini R, et al. New laser Doppler scanner, a valuable adjunct in burn depth assessment. Burns 1993;19(6):485–9.
18. Claes KEY, Hoeksema H, Robbens C, et al. The LDI Enigma, Part I: so much proof, so little use. Burns 2021;47(8):1783–92.
19. Claes KEY, Hoeksema H, Robbens C, et al. The LDI Enigma Part II: indeterminate depth burns, man or machine? Burns 2021;47(8):1773–82.
20. Asif M, Chin AGM, Lagziel T, et al. The added benefit of combining laser Doppler imaging with clinical evaluation in determining the need for excision of indeterminate-depth burn wounds. Cureus 2020;12(6):e8774.
21. Asuku M, Yu TC, Yan Q, et al. Split-thickness skin graft donor-site morbidity: a systematic literature review. Burns 2021;47(7):1525–46.
22. Rowland R, Ponticorvo A, Baldado M, et al. Burn wound classification model using spatial frequency-domain imaging and machine learning. J Biomed Opt 2019;24(5):1–9.
23. Ponticorvo A, Rowland R, Baldado M, et al. Spatial Frequency Domain Imaging (SFDI) of clinical burns: a case report. Burns Open 2020;4(2):67–71.
24. Yin M, Li Y, Luo Y, et al. A novel method for objectively, rapidly and accurately evaluating burn depth via near infrared spectroscopy. Burns Trauma 2021;9:tkab014.
25. Jaskille AD, Shupp JW, Jordan MH, et al. Critical review of burn depth assessment techniques: Part I. Historical review. J Burn Care Res 2009; 30(6):937–47.
26. Smart C. On burns by gunpowder and scalds by steam. Lancet 1876;2:421–2.
27. Schjerning OV. About the death as a result of burning and scalding from the court physician standpoint. 1884;41(24-66):273-300.
28. Meeh K. Surface measurements of the human body. Z Biol 1879;15:425–58.
29. Weidenfeld S, Zumbusch LV. More contributions to pathology and therapy of severe burns. Arch Dermatol Syph 1905;163–87.
30. Du Bois D, Du Bois EF. A formula to estimate the approximate surface area if height and weight be known. 1916. Nutrition 1989;5(5):303–11. discussion 312-3.
31. Murari A, Singh KN. Lund and Browder chart-modified versus original: a comparative study. Acute Crit Care 2019;34(4):276–81.
32. Wallace AB. The exposure treatment of burns. Lancet 1951;1(6653):501–4.
33. Rashaan ZM, Euser AM, van Zuijlen PPM, et al. Three-dimensional imaging is a novel and reliable technique to measure total body surface area. Burns 2018;44(4):816–22.
34. Williams RY, Wohlgemuth SD. Does the "rule of nines" apply to morbidly obese burn victims? J Burn Care Res 2013;34(4):447–52.
35. Choi J, Patil A, Vendrow E, et al. Practical computer vision application to compute total body surface

area burn: reappraising a fundamental burn injury formula in the modern era. JAMA Surg 2022; 157(2):129–35.

36. Underhill FP. The significance of anhydremia in extensive surface burns. JAMA 1930;95(12):852–7.

37. Cope O, Moore FD. The redistribution of body water and the fluid therapy of the burned patient. Ann Surg 1947;126(6):1010–45.

38. Pruitt BA Jr, Wolf SE. An historical perspective on advances in burn care over the past 100 years. Clin Plast Surg 2009;36(4):527–45.

39. Moore FD. The body-weight burn budget. Basic fluid therapy for the early burn. Surg Clin North Am 1970;50(6):1249–65.

40. Evans EI, Purnell OJ, Robinett PW, et al. Fluid and electrolyte requirements in severe burns. Ann Surg 1952;135(6):804–17.

41. Baxter CR, Shires T. Physiological response to crystalloid resuscitation of severe burns. Ann N Y Acad Sci 1968;150(3):874–94.

42. Barillo DJ. Topical antimicrobials in burn wound care: a recent history. Wounds. Jul 2008;20(7): 192–8.

43. Haller JS Jr. Treatment of infected wounds during the great war, 1914 to 1918. South Med J 1992; 85(3):303–15.

44. Heggers JP, Sazy JA, Stenberg BD, et al. Bactericidal and wound-healing properties of sodium hypochlorite solutions: the 1991 Lindberg Award. J Burn Care Rehabil 1991;12(5):420–4.

45. Pruskowski KA, Mitchell TA, Kiley JL, et al. Diagnosis and management of invasive fungal wound infections in burn patients. European Burn Journal 2021;2(4):168–83.

46. Lindberg RB, Moncrief JA, Switzer WE, et al. The successful control of burn wound sepsis. J Trauma 1965;5(5):601–16.

47. Cancio LC. Topical antimicrobial agents for burn wound care: history and current status. Surg Infect (Larchmt) 2021;22(1):3–11.

48. Fox CL Jr. Silver sulfadiazine–a new topical therapy for Pseudomonas in burns. Therapy of Pseudomonas infection in burns. Arch Surg 1968;96(2): 184–8.

49. Moyer CA, Brentano L, Gravens DL, et al. Treatment of large human burns with 0.5 per cent silver nitrate solution. Arch Surg 1965;90:812–67.

50. Burke JF, Quinby WC, Bondoc CC, et al. The contribution of a bacterially isolated environment to the prevention of infection in seriously burned patients. Ann Surg 1977;186(3):377–87.

51. Bang RL, Sharma PN, Sanyal SC, et al. ticaemia after burn injury: a comparative study. Burns 2002; 28(8):746–51.

52. Ozhathil DK, Tay MW, Wolf SE, Branski LK. A Narrative Review of the History of Skin Grafting in Burn Care. Medicina (Kaunas) 2021;57(4):380.

53. Hauben DJ, Baruchin A, Mahler A. On the history of the free skin graft. Ann Plast Surg 1982;9(3):242–5.

54. Warren JM. Taliacotian operation. Boston Med Surg J 1840;22:261–9.

55. Singh M, Nuutila K, Collins KC, et al. Evolution of skin grafting for treatment of burns: Reverdin pinch grafting to Tanner mesh grafting and beyond. Burns 2017;43(6):1149–54.

56. Ehrenfried A. Reverdin and other methods of skingrafting: historical. Boston Med Surg J 1909; 161(26):911–7.

57. Ameer F, Singh AK, Kumar S. Evolution of instruments for harvest of the skin grafts. Indian J Plast Surg 2013;46(1):28–35.

58. Liu HF, Zhang F, Lineaweaver WC. History and advancement of burn treatments. Ann Plast Surg. Feb 2017;78(2 Suppl 1):S2–8.

59. Cope O, Langohr JL, Moore FD, Webster RC. Expeditious Care of Full-Thickness Burn Wounds by Surgical Excision and Grafting. Ann Surg 1947;125(1):1–22.

60. Jackson D, Topley E, Cason JS, et al. Primary excision and grafting of large burns. Ann Surg 1960; 152(2):167–89.

61. Janzekovic Z. A new concept in the early excision and immediate grafting of burns. J Trauma 1970; 10(12):1103–8.

62. Monafo WW. Tangential excision. Clin Plast Surg 1974;1(4):591–601.

63. Burke JF, Bondoc CC, Quinby WC. Primary burn excision and immediate grafting: a method shortening illness. J Trauma. May 1974;14(5):389–95.

64. Tompkins RG, Remensnyder JP, Burke JF, et al. Significant reductions in mortality for children with burn injuries through the use of prompt eschar excision. Ann Surg. Nov 1988;208(5):577–85.

65. Herndon DN, Barrow RE, Rutan RL, et al. A comparison of conservative versus early excision. Therapies in severely burned patients. Ann Surg. May 1989;209(5):547–52. discussion 552-3.

66. Xiao-Wu W, Herndon DN, Spies M, et al. Effects of delayed wound excision and grafting in severely burned children. Arch Surg 2002;137(9):1049–54.

67. De Decker I, De Graeve L, Hoeksema H, et al. Enzymatic debridement: past, present, and future. Acta Chir Belg 2022;122(4):279–95.

68. Heitzmann W, Fuchs PC, Schiefer JL. Historical Perspectives on the Development of Current Standards of Care for Enzymatic Debridement. Medicina (Kaunas) 2020;56(12):706.

69. Garret TA. Bacillus subtilis protease: a new topical agent for debridement. Clin Med 1969;76:11–5.

70. Hirche C, Kreken Almeland S, Dheansa B, et al. Eschar removal by bromelain based enzymatic debridement (Nexobrid(R)) in burns: European consensus guidelines update. Burns 2020;46(4): 782–96.

71. Bondoc CC, Burke JF. Clinical experience with viable frozen human skin and a frozen skin bank. Ann Surg 1971;174(3):371–82.

72. Heimbach D, Luterman A, Burke J, et al. Artificial dermis for major burns. A multi-center randomized clinical trial. Ann Surg Sep 1988;208(3):313–20.

73. Haddad AG, Giatsidis G, Orgill DP, et al. Skin substitutes and bioscaffolds: temporary and permanent coverage. Clin Plast Surg. Jul 2017;44(3):627–34.

74. Robinson DH, Toledo AH. Historical development of modern anesthesia. J Invest Surg 2012;25(3):141–9.

75. Borges AF. Elective incisions and scar revision. Boston: Little Brown & Co. Inc.; 1973.

76. Robson MC, Koss N, Krizek TJ, et al. The undelayed Mutter flap in head and neck reconstruction. Am J Surg 1976;132(4):472–5.

77. Davis JS. The relaxation of scar contractures by means of the Z-or reversed Z-type incision: stressing the use of scar infiltrated tissues. Ann Surg. Nov 1931;94(5):871–84.

78. Webster JP. The early history of the tubed pedicle flap. Surg Clin North Am. Apr 1959;39(2):261–75.

79. Kantar RS, Alfonso AR, Diep GK, et al. Facial transplantation: principles and evolving concepts. Plast Reconstr Surg 2021;147(6):1022e–38e.

80. Spetz J. Chapter 3: Physicians and Physicists, The interdisciplinary introduction of the laser to medicine. In: Rosenberg N, Gelijns AC, Dawkins H, editors. Sources of medical technology: universities and industry. Washington, DC: National Academies Press; 1995. p. 41–66.

81. Alster TS. Improvement of erythematous and hypertrophic scars by the 585-nm flashlamp-pumped pulsed dye laser. Ann Plast Surg 1994;32(2):186–90.

82. Anderson RR, Parrish JA. Selective photothermolysis: precise microsurgery by selective absorption of pulsed radiation. Science. Apr 29 1983;220(4596):524–7.

83. Manstein D, Herron GS, Sink RK, et al. Fractional photothermolysis: a new concept for cutaneous remodeling using microscopic patterns of thermal injury. Lasers Surg Med 2004;34(5):426–38.

84. Donelan MB, Parrett BM, Sheridan RL. Pulsed dye laser therapy and z-plasty for facial burn scars: the alternative to excision. Ann Plast Surg. May 2008;60(5):480–6.

85. Wenande E, Anderson RR, Haedersdal M. Fundamentals of fractional laser-assisted drug delivery: an in-depth guide to experimental methodology and data interpretation. Adv Drug Deliv Rev 2020;153:169–84.

86. Issler-Fisher AC, Waibel JS, Donelan MB. Laser modulation of hypertrophic scars: technique and practice. Clin Plast Surg 2017;44(4):757–66.

87. Choi KJ, Williams EA, Pham CH, et al. Fractional CO(2) laser treatment for burn scar improvement: a systematic review and meta-analysis. Burns 2021;47(2):259–69.

88. Klifto KM, Asif M, Hultman CS. Laser management of hypertrophic burn scars: a comprehensive review. Burns Trauma 2020;8:tkz002.

89. Miletta N, Siwy K, Hivnor C, et al. Fractional ablative laser therapy is an effective treatment for hypertrophic burn scars: a prospective study of objective and subjective outcomes. Ann Surg 2021;274(6):e574–80.

90. Turk JL. Inflammation: John Hunter's "A treatise on the blood, inflammation and gun-shot wounds". Int J Exp Pathol 1994;75(6):385–95.

91. Reiss E, Pearson E, Artz CP. The metabolic response to burns. J Clin Invest 1956;35(1):62–77.

92. Newsome TW, Mason AD Jr, Pruitt BA Jr. Weight loss following thermal injury. Ann Surg 1973;178(2):215–7.

93. Cuthbertson DP. Second annual Jonathan E. Rhoads Lecture. The metabolic response to injury and its nutritional implications: retrospect and prospect. JPEN J Parenter Enteral Nutr May-Jun 1979;3(3):108–29.

94. Wilmore DW, Long JM, Mason AD Jr, et al. Catecholamines: mediator of the hypermetabolic response to thermal injury. Ann Surg 1974;180(4):653–69.

95. Bessey PQ, Watters JM, Aoki TT, et al. Combined hormonal infusion simulates the metabolic response to injury. Ann Surg 1984;200(3):264–81.

96. Shaffer PA, Coleman W. Protein metabolism in typhoid fever. Arch Intern Med 1909;IV(6):538–600.

97. Wilmore DW, Curreri PW, Spitzer KW, et al. Supranormal dietary intake in thermally injured hypermetabolic patients. Surg Gynecol Obstet 1971;132:881–6.

98. Curreri PW, Richmond D, Marvin J, et al. Dietary requirements of patients with major burns. J Am Diet Assoc 1974;65(4):415–7.

99. Herndon DN, Barrow RE, Stein M, et al. Increased mortality with intravenous supplemental feeding in severely burned patients. J Burn Care Rehabil 1989;10(4):309–13.

100. Herndon DN, Hart DW, Wolf SE, et al. Reversal of catabolism by beta-blockade after severe burns. N Engl J Med 2001;345(17):1223–9.

101. Ramzy PI, Wolf SE, Herndon DN. Current status of anabolic hormone administration in human burn injury. JPEN J Parenter Enteral Nutr 1999;23(6 Suppl):S190–4.

102. Cioffi WG, Gore DC, Rue LW 3rd, et al. Insulin-like growth factor-1 lowers protein oxidation in patients with thermal injury. Ann Surg 1994;220(3):310–6. discussion 316-9.

103. Diaz EC, Herndon DN, Porter C, et al. Effects of pharmacological interventions on muscle protein synthesis and breakdown in recovery from burns. Burns 2015;41(4):649–57.

104. Jeschke MG, Finnerty CC, Kulp GA, et al. Combination of recombinant human growth hormone and propranolol decreases hypermetabolism and inflammation in severely burned children. Pediatr Crit Care Med 2008;9(2):209–16.

105. Thomas SJ, Morimoto K, Herndon DN, et al. The effect of prolonged euglycemic hyperinsulinemia on lean body mass after severe burn. Surgery 2002; 132(2):341–7.

106. Ring J, Heinelt M, Sharma S, et al. Oxandrolone in the treatment of burn injuries: a systematic review and meta-analysis. J Burn Care Res 2020;41(1):190–9.

107. Foley FD, Moncrief JA, Mason AD Jr. Pathology of the lung in fatally burned patints. Ann Surg. Feb 1968;167(2):251–64.

108. Moylan JA, Chan CK. Inhalation injury–an increasing problem. Ann Surg. Jul 1978;188(1):34–7.

109. Hunt JL, Agee RN, Pruitt BA Jr. Fiberoptic bronchoscopy in acute inhalation injury. J Trauma 1975;15(8):641–9.

110. Agee RN, Long JM 3rd, Hunt JL, et al. Use of 133xenon in early diagnosis of inhalation injury. J Trauma 1976;16(3):218–24.

111. Moylan JA Jr, Wilmore DW, Mouton DE, et al. Early diagnosis of inhalation injury using 133 xenon lung scan. Ann Surg 1972;176(4):477–84.

112. Shirani KZ, Pruitt BA Jr, Mason AD Jr. The influence of inhalation injury and pneumonia on burn mortality. Ann Surg 1987;205(1):82–7.

113. Cioffi WG Jr, Rue LW 3rd, Graves TA, et al. Prophylactic use of high-frequency percussive ventilation in patients with inhalation injury. Ann Surg 1991; 213(6):575–80. discussion 580-2.

114. Wood FM. The role of cell-based therapies in acute burn wound skin repair: a review. J Burn Care Res 2023;44(Suppl_1):S42–7.

115. Henriksen JL, Sørensen NB, Fink T, et al. Systematic Review of Stem-Cell-Based Therapy of Burn Wounds: Lessons Learned from Animal and Clinical Studies. Cells 2020;9(12):2545.

116. Cohen BP, Bernstein JL, Morrison KA, et al. Tissue engineering the human auricle by auricular chondrocyte-mesenchymal stem cell co-implantation. PLoS One 2018;13(10):e0202356.

117. Wang H, Wang Z, Liu H, et al. Three-Dimensional printing strategies for irregularly shaped cartilage tissue engineering: current state and challenges. Front Bioeng Biotechnol 2022;9:777039.

118. Stewart BT, Nsaful K, Allorto N, et al. Burn care in low-resource and austere settings. Surg Clin North Am 2023;103(3):551–63.

119. James SL, Lucchesi LR, Bisignano C, et al. Epidemiology of injuries from fire, heat and hot substances: global, regional and national morbidity and mortality estimates from the Global Burden of Disease 2017 study. Inj Prev 2020;26(Suppl 2): i36–45.

Fluid Resuscitation and Cardiovascular Support in Acute Burn Care

Zachary J. Collier, MD, MS[a], Justin Gillenwater, MD, MS[a,b],*

KEYWORDS

• Fluid resuscitation • Acute burn management • Burn shock • Crystalloid • Colloid • Critical care

KEY POINTS

- The systemic inflammatory response caused by large burns requires resuscitation to maintain tissue perfusion.
- While the endpoints of resuscitation are still debated, the mean arterial pressure and hourly urine output remain standard markers for adequate perfusion in most patients.
- Newer technologies may lead to improvements in guided resuscitation, but their use is not yet widespread. More research is required to validate their use in patients with burns.

INTRODUCTION

This article reviews the underlying pathophysiology of burn injury which necessitates fluid resuscitation and discusses a suggested algorithm for restoring normal fluid balance during the acute burn phase. As with many core areas of critical care medicine, there exist much data, which have created consensus on general points although some controversies remain. Throughout the discussion of this topic, it is important to remember that each patient and their injuries are unique. Therefore, it is valuable to understand the core concepts while simultaneously tailoring treatment for each specific patient to achieve best results.

PATHOPHYSIOLOGY
Overview

Burn injury causes local and systemic changes that must be considered during the initial evaluation and stabilization of acute injuries. Large burns (>20% total body surface area [TBSA]) result in release of inflammatory mediators from damaged tissue that can exert their effects on the body causing a variety of derangements across numerous organ systems. Predictable alterations of major organ systems are the result, leading to hypovolemic shock followed by multiple organ system dysfunction should the appropriate interventions be delayed or incomplete.

During the first 24 hours following a massive burn, increased vascular permeability leads to egress of water from the vascular to the interstitial space. This decreases the available intravascular fluid volume, which necessitates replacement to ensure adequate end-organ perfusion. If intravascular losses are not adequately repleted, there is generalized and organ-specific hypoperfusion. Cardiac output (CO) is diminished because of fluid shifts and changes in systemic vascular resistance as a catecholamine surge occurs at significant levels. Gastrointestinal and renal systems are the first to exhibit dysfunction but eventually all organ systems may become impacted. Electrolyte imbalances are common and intercellular ion shifts occur from cellular death in damaged tissues. Endocrine function is decreased, insulin and cortisol requirements increase, and hyperglycemia

[a] Division of Plastic & Reconstructive Surgery, USC Department of Surgery, University of Chicago, 1510 San Pablo Street, Suite 415, Los Angeles, CA 90033, USA; [b] Plastic and Reconstructive Surgery, University of Southern California
* Corresponding author. Southern California Regional Burn Center at LAC+USC, IPT - Burn Unit 5D & 5M, Room. 5G113A, 2051 Marengo Street, Los Angeles, CA 90033.
E-mail address: justin.gillenwater@med.usc.edu

Clin Plastic Surg 51 (2024) 205–220
https://doi.org/10.1016/j.cps.2023.10.003
0094-1298/24/© 2023 Elsevier Inc. All rights reserved.

is common. The initial massive inflammatory response is subsequently followed by a period of immunosuppression. As a result, effective therapeutic interventions require an intimate knowledge of the physiologic changes that occur both locally and systemically.

Local Response: Burn Wound Edema and Tissue Loss

Thermal, chemical, and radiation-induced injury to the skin results in cell death through a variety of mechanisms including coagulation, protein denaturation, and cell rupture. Cellular injury and death cause the release of many inflammatory mediators, such as histamine, bradykinin, and prostaglandins. These mediators act locally to create tissue edema by altering connections in the basement membrane and increasing endothelial cell permeability. This results in transudation of large, osmotically active intravascular proteins out of the capillaries and into the interstitium of burned tissues.[1,2] Plasma oncotic pressure is reduced and causes water to follow the oncotic gradient from the microvascular capillary circulation into burned tissue to create edema. Additionally, interstitial hydrostatic pressure is increased as integrins are broken and cell-to-cell adhesion is disrupted.[2] This leads to exposure of hydrophilic proteoglycans, which further drives water into the interstitial space. The summation of these interactions leads to profound and immediate edema in burn-injured tissue, which can also expand outside of the initial burn area to create similar edema elsewhere in the region and potentially systemically should the burn injury be large enough to release a sufficient amount of tissue factor and inflammatory mediators.

In addition, tissue injury leads to the release of endogenous damage-associated molecular patterns (DAMPs) like mitochondrial DNA which is recognized via pattern recognition receptors (eg, Toll-like receptors [TLRs], NOD-like receptors [NLRs]) and stimulates the release of cytokines, such as interleukin-1 (IL-1), interleukin-8 (IL-8), and tumor necrosis factor-alpha (TNFα).[3] This attracts leukocytes to the wound resulting in neutrophil degranulation that releases proteases and generates reactive oxygen species, which further damages surrounding tissues. Although this response acts as a useful microbicide in smaller burns, this process is cytotoxic to normal tissue when larger burn areas are involved. The complement system is also activated, particularly in burns greater than 20% TBSA, which disrupts dermal microvasculature through thrombosis to perpetuate local tissue ischemia and necrosis.[4–6]

Systemic Response: Burn Shock and Burn Edema

Burns greater than 20% of TBSA cause a system-wide inflammatory response.[7] The large surge of inflammatory mediators and cytokines into the circulation causes leaky microvasculature, vasodilation, and decreased CO. With increasing burn size, the growing magnitude of the local response creates a spillover effect from the microenvironment to the entire system.

As in burned tissue, capillary integrity becomes compromised systemically due to circulating cytokines and alarmins. The low-flow state coupled with an osmotic and oncotic pressure graduate generated by transudate of proteins and electrolytes results in a profound efflux of intravascular volume into the interstitial space. Hematocrit increases as intravascular volume rapidly decreases, and along with complement activation, creates a hypercoagulable state. Changes in cell membrane integrity cause additional sequestration of fluid within the intracellular space that propagates cellular-level injury. The aggregate effect of these processes causes a rapid onset total body edema with maximal fluid shifts occurring around 12 hours postburn.[8,9]

In contrast to burned tissue, capillary integrity in non-burned tissue returns to near normal within 24 hours, and transudation of colloids out of the vascular space decreases.[10] However, water continues to collect in the interstitial space in non-burned tissue even after capillary integrity has been restored because of loss of normal oncotic gradient. The loss of plasma proteins into burned tissue is significant enough to decrease vascular oncotic pressure, resulting in ongoing third spacing of water throughout the body.

Predicting and compensating for intravascular volume loss is further complicated by the fact that large burns result in significant insensible heat and water losses that further exacerbate the previously discussed causes of hypovolemia. With the loss of the body's natural barrier that facilitates water and temperature regulation, the subsequent evaporative losses and hypothermia both directly and indirectly worsen the hypovolemic state. The evaporative losses allow the already increasing third space phenomenon to worsen as the evaporation drives extravascular water gradient. Hypothermia may also lead to blood loss as the resulting dysfunction in platelet aggregation allows for greater blood loss from external and internal wounds.[11]

Burn shock is multifactorial because of the interplay between loss of intravascular volume, cardiac dysfunction, hypercoagulability, insensible losses, hypothermia, and vascular changes (**Fig. 1**).

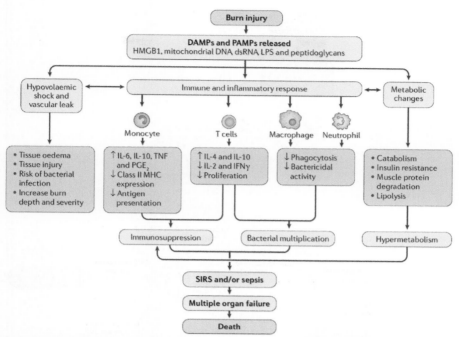

Fig. 1. Overview of burn pathophysiology. (*From*: Jeschke MG, van Baar ME, Choudhry MA, Chung KK, Gibran NS, Logsetty S. Burn injury. Nat Rev Dis Primer. 2020;6(1):11. https://doi.org/10.1038/s41572-020-0145-5)

Although hypovolemia is a primary driver of shock during the early phase of acute burn injury, vasodilation also develops due to the massive release of inflammatory mediators exacerbating the volume-based shock. The resultant shock from hypovolemia and vasodilation seen in large burns is further compounded by cardiac contractile dysfunction.[12] Cardiac dysfunction can arise primarily from contractility deficits triggered by massive cytokine releases or secondarily from decreased circulating blood volume due to serum loss.[13] These changes in pre-load, contractility, and after-load may act independently or in concert to cause low CO and resultant end-organ hypoperfusion.

While cardiovascular collapse may happen early in burn shock due to the aforementioned reasons, renal failure often happens in close proximity due to the subsequent hypoperfusion of these very sensitive, flow-dependent organs.[14,15] Increased blood viscosity from the elevated hematocrit and myoglobinemia from deeper tissue damage coupled with depleted intravascular volume leads to poor perfusion and acute renal failure. Given that urine output is a primary endpoint for guiding resuscitation, it is essential that renal function is preserved early on during the resuscitative efforts to ensure that ongoing fluid management is both timely and effective.

While end-organ hypoperfusion is most immediately recognizable with critical organs such as the

heart and kidneys, burn shock has a great impact on the burn injury itself. The injured tissue within the "zone of stasis," which is like the penumbra or watershed area of a stroke, experiences malperfusion and subsequently converts to the "zone of coagulation" or irreversible damage.[16,17]

RESUSCITATION

The main objective for treating acute burn shock is to provide supportive care with fluid resuscitation until vascular permeability is restored and interstitial fluid losses are overcome. Accomplishing this requires interventions to facilitate end-organ perfusion while limiting fluid overload. Over-resuscitation has undesirable sequelae, such as conversion of partial thickness burns to full thickness, pulmonary edema, and abdominal compartment syndrome.[10,18–20] There is ongoing debate about the optimal fluid for resuscitation, the timing of fluid administration, the volume of fluid to administer, the impact of age on fluid requirements, the adjustments needed for inhalation injury, and the way in which different burn mechanisms impact fluid requirements. Similarly, precise end points of resuscitation are controversial, particularly due to the impact of the burn shock on the reliability of such measurements. However, 2 guiding principles are clear. First, resuscitation should involve the least amount of fluid necessary

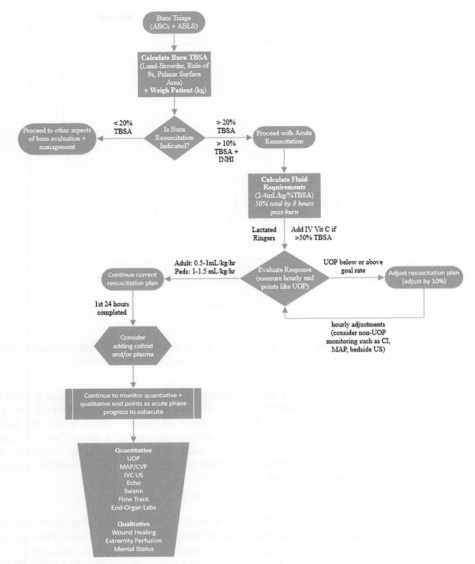

Fig. 2. Fluid resuscitation pathway.

to provide organ perfusion. Second, the resuscitation should be continuously adjusted to prevent over-resuscitation (ie, fluid creep) and under-resuscitation (**Fig. 2**).[5,21]

Two determinants that guide initial efforts at resuscitation are the size of the burn (ie, TBSA) and the size of the person (ie, kg) burned. The larger the burn, the larger the person, the more fluid needed to resuscitate.[22] Multiple formulas have been adopted which use these 2 variables; the Parkland formula being the most popular. Using this formula, fluid needs are estimated at 4 mL/kg/% TBSA burn for the first 24 hours, with half of the total volume given within the first 8 hours and the remaining half over the subsequent 16 hours.[21]

Lactated Ringer (LR) solution is the crystalloid of choice using this formula.[19] Other formulas with increasing application are the modified Brooke formula and consensus formulas (**Table 1**) which are crystalloid-based resuscitations that advocate 2 and 3 mL/kg/% TBSA, respectively. As resuscitation efforts proceed, the rate of fluid given is titrated based on predetermined end points. In our center, the authors begin with the modified Brooke formula and adjust fluid rates using vital signs, such as mean arterial pressures (MAP) and hourly urine output (UOP), with goal UOP between 0.5 and 1 mL/kg in adults or 1 to 1.5 mL/kg in children under 18 years. Strictly adhering to any of the aforementioned formulas may result in under-

Table 1
Abls fluid resuscitation guidelines

Burn Type	Age & Weight	Adjusted Fluid Rate
Flame or Scald	Adults + children ≥ 14 years old Children < 14 years old Infants + children ≤ 30 kg	2 mL LR × kg × % TBSA 3 mL LR × kg × % TBSA 3 mL LR × kg × % TBSA *Plus D5 LR at maintenance rate*
Electricity injury	All ages	4 mL LR × kg × % TBSA *Plus D5 LR at maintenance rate for infants and young children*

Advanced Burn Life Support™ Manual, 2023. Reprinted (in part) with permission from American Burn Association. Copyright© 2023 American Burn Association: https://ameriburn.org/abls.

resuscitation or over-resuscitation, so close monitoring of patient-specific response to fluids is critical for successful implementation.

Alternate forms of monitoring in addition to simply measuring UOP may lend to improved resuscitative efforts and are discussed later.[22–24] Larger burn size, depth of burn, and presence of inhalational injury have also all been correlated with fluid requirements greater than predicted by the Parkland formula.[25,26]

Other formulas that guide resuscitation are described, some incorporating the use of colloids and/or plasma. The debate on crystalloids versus colloids is as old as the history of burn care. Although arguments are made to support either position, the supporting evidence is contradictory, and no consensus recommendation exists.

Crystalloid Alone

Crystalloid-only resuscitation is commonly used by burn providers as it is inexpensive, readily available, and has a proven track record. Physiologically, capillaries in burned tissue remain leaky for more than 48 hours, which means that theoretically any colloids being infused during that time would continue to leak into the burned tissue. This ongoing extravascular leakage further perpetuates the osmotic drive of water to migrate into the interstitial space which worsens edema. This theoretic risk deters many burn providers from utilizing colloid and using crystalloid-only paradigms. Although logical, this thesis has not been proven to occur in human burn tissue. There is no consensus statement regarding appropriate choice of crystalloid, but the most common is Lactated Ringer's (LR) solution, which is a balanced crystalloid providing 130 mEq/L of sodium, 4 mEq of potassium, and 28 mEq of lactate. LR is hypo-osmolar in comparison to serum plasma, but it is effective at restoring extracellular sodium deficits.[27] The sodium lactate in the solution is metabolized by the liver to bicarbonate and thus the solution is alkalinizing. It is important to note that the sodium lactate is not the same as the lactic acid which contributes to metabolic acidosis, and LR does not contribute to or worsen such acidoses.[28] On the contrary, normal saline (0.9% NS) with 154 mEq of sodium and 154 mEq of chloride induces academia because of the dissociation of these ions in solution. In the setting of the lactic acidosis that accompanies burn injuries, this is undesirable and can potentiate the acidosis rather than correct it. As a result, our burn unit uses LR for crystalloid resuscitation and avoids normal saline. In the setting of hyperkalemia, sodium bicarbonate solution may be used but research shows that the 4 mEq of potassium in LR cannot worsen or potentiate hyperkalemia.[28]

Hypertonic Saline

Hypertonic (3%) saline is a largely historic alternative to traditional crystalloid. In theory, hypertonic saline acts osmotically to draw water from the interstitium into the intravascular space, thereby lessening fluid requirements. First popularized in the 1970s for use in the burn population, its use has been shown to reduce the amount of volume needed to maintain a target UOP.[29] More recent reports suggest that increasing the intravascular osmolality by using hypertonic saline limits edema formation and reduces the incidence of abdominal compartment syndrome.[18] Other authors, however, have reported that hypertonic saline does not reduce total fluid loads.

Alarmingly, studies have also associated increased incidence of hypernatremia, renal failure, and mortality when hypertonic saline was used in burn resuscitation.[30,31] Given these potentially devastating consequences, it is our opinion that hypertonic saline solutions have no role in the resuscitation of the burned patient and their use should be avoided. Due to similar concerns, despite initially suggesting a benefit to such hypertonic solutions, Monafo later in 1996 recommended not using hypertonic as a burn resuscitation fluid (**Table 2**).[32]

Table 2
Intravenous fluid compositions versus plasma

| Solute | Plasma | Colloids | | | Crystalloids | |
		Dextran	Gelatin	Normal Saline (0.9%)	Lactated Ringers (LR)	Plasma Lyte
Na$^+$	135–145	154	154	154	130	140
K$^+$	4.0–5.0	0	0	0	4	5
Ca^{2+}	2.2–2.6	0	0	0	2.7	0
Mg^{2+}	1.0–2.0	0	0	0	0	1.5
Cl$^-$	95–110	154	120	154	109	98
Acetate	0	0	0	0	0	27
Lactate	0.8–1.8	0	0	0	28	0
Gluconate	0	0	0	0	0	23
Bicarbonate	23–26	0	0	0	0	0
Osmolarity	291	308	274	308	280	294
Colloid	35–45	100	40	0	0	0
pH	7.4	-	-	5.7	6.5	7.4

Abbreviations: Ca, calcium; Cl, chloride; K, potassium; Mg, magnesium; Na, sodium.
Osmolarity (mOsm/L); colloid (g/L); other solutes (mmol/L).

Colloids and Starches

The use of colloids, starches, and plasma in burn resuscitation remains controversial but growing data support a place for these resuscitative methods. Proponents of colloids assert that these fluids are osmotically active intravascularly, require less volume to achieve a given end point, and may lead to less edema.[33–36] In theory, the capillary beds in non-burned tissue return to baseline levels of permeability at 5 to 8 hours after initial thermal injury.[37] Resuscitation after this time with colloids, such as albumin, fresh frozen plasma (FFP), or long chain polysaccharides, could provide circulating intravascular volume and lessen fluid needs.[38,39] Decreased fluid volumes during initial resuscitation would lead to less global tissue edema and therefore decreased risks of compartment syndromes or other sequelae of over-resuscitation.

The evidence for use of albumin or other colloids in burn resuscitation is plentiful and many burn institutions use them regularly in their resuscitation protocols. In a retrospective study, albumin use has been linked with decreased mortality when controlling for age, burn size, and inhalational injury.[33] In another retrospective study specific to patients with large burns, albumin use has been demonstrated to decrease the incidence of extremity compartment syndrome and renal failure.[30] A recent meta-analysis of albumin use in acute burn resuscitation found that its use was associated with decreased mortality and decreased incidence of compartment syndrome.[40] When determining which patients may benefit from albumin during the initial resuscitation, a recent study called the Acute Burn ResUscitation Multicenter Prospective Trial (ABRUPT) showed that patients who received albumin were most likely to have had poor initial responses to crystalloid (ie, higher than calculated to achieve end point goals), be older in age, have greater TBSA and burn depth, and early signs of organ failure.[41]

A prospective, randomized trial, comparing the use of LR alone against LR and FFP demonstrated that use of FFP was correlated with nearly 50% less total volume used compared to the crystalloid-only group and that patients had lower intraabdominal pressures as well as faster clearance of the base deficit.[42] Another study out of Turkey in patients with over 30% TBSA burns found that the mortality rate in the plasma-based resuscitation group was less than half that of the colloid-based group (34% vs 79%).[43] Two other studies looking at early administration of FFP during the first 12 hours of admission found that patients who received FFP had greater UOP with reduced total fluid requirements while there were no reported cases of transfusion-related acute lung injury , acute coronary syndrome, acute respiratory distress syndrome, or acute kidney injury.[44,45] With recent advances in the processing and storage of FFP as well as a greater understanding of when and for whom to transfuse, the role of FFP in acute burn resuscitation protocols is becoming increasingly and more broadly accepted.

However, the evidence against the use of colloids is equally plentiful. Cochrane systematic reviews have concluded that in resuscitation of critically ill patients, there is no improvement in mortality when using colloids over crystalloids alone.[36] Similarly, there is no difference in outcomes among the various colloid solutions.[46,47] Moreover, in burned patients, colloid use has been associated with increased lung water after finishing resuscitation.[34] A double blind, randomized clinical trial has demonstrated that hydroxyethyl starch is not superior to LR alone.[35] FFP can cause transfusion-associated lung injury and allergic and anaphylactic reactions, so these risks must be weight against the previously mentioned benefits.

Given that colloids are more expensive and may have drawbacks when compared with iso-osmotic crystalloid solutions alone, the clinician should be judicious in their use. They may have a role in the patient with fluid-sensitive comorbidities, such as in chronic renal or heart failure as well as those who fail to respond to crystalloid resuscitation.

In authors' burn unit, albumin is used during resuscitation in 2 situations: (1) symptomatic low oncotic pressure after massive crystalloid resuscitation, and (2) when resuscitation is failing to support end-organ perfusion with clinical end points. With massive burn injuries, the volume of crystalloid needed to maintain tissue perfusion predictably dilutes the albumin remaining in the intravascular space. The result is an imbalance between intravascular and extracellular oncotic and hydrostatic pressures. This leads to ongoing loss of intravascular volume and excessive resuscitation. Depending on the patient, this occurs when albumin levels drop lower than 1.2 to 1.5 g/dL. In some patients with serious burns, standard Parkland formula resuscitation is not successful. In many patients, the use of a 5% albumin solution results in restoration of effective perfusion.[1] Although the mechanistic rationale for this treatment is not known, senior members of the burn community supported this algorithm at the National Institutes of Health state of the art consensus conference (Table 3).

Adjuncts to Resuscitation

The massive inflammatory reaction to burn injury is acknowledged by all. A component of this is neutrophil degranulation, which releases large qualities of oxygen free radicals. Some have proposed this as a mechanism for burn wound progression even in well-resuscitated patients. Antioxidants could therefore play a role in decreasing the effect of reactive oxygen species in burned tissue. The data for use of ascorbic acid (vitamin C) are clear in experimental models and are suggestive enough to support its use in the acutely burned patient.[48] High-dose ascorbic acid delivered during the first 24 hours after a large burn has been shown to reduce fluid volume needed for adequate resuscitation.[49,50] A more recent meta-analysis that included 16 studies and 924 patients using high-dose vitamin C (66 mg/kg/hr) found 30% to 50% reductions in total fluid requirements, decreased time to wound healing (2.5–10 days faster), and a 10% to 20% lower mortality rate.[51] Although administration of vitamin C has reportedly been complicated by oxalate nephropathy,[52] the authors believe the evidence is sufficient to recommend the use of ascorbic acid as an adjunct to resuscitation.

Other important supplements to fluid resuscitation, particularly in the critically ill burn patient, are vasoactive medications which encompass a broad range of agents (Table 4) that act on various aspects of the cardiovascular system. Careful selection of these agents will help critical care providers to manipulate cardiac inotropy and systemic vascular resistance, which will subsequently alter cardiac output and blood pressure. These agents act on a variety of receptors including alpha-1, beta-1 and -2, dopamine-1 and -2, and vasopressin-1 and -2. A detailed summary of the various vasoactive agents, their receptor targets, and impact on the cardiovascular system is provided in Table 4. Utilization of both traditional and newer monitoring methods (discussed below) is essential for the initial selection and subsequent titration of vasoactive agents to ensure cardiac output is optimized while end point perfusion is maintained. Knowing when, why, and how to implement these important adjuncts are central to the burn specialist's expertise.

MONITORING AND END POINTS TO RESUSCITATION

Monitoring of the patient with large burns is critical to determine end points of resuscitation. Assessing end-organ perfusion is accomplished using clinical, hemodynamic, renal, and biochemical parameters, which guide dynamic resuscitative efforts. Outcomes are improved when resuscitation is guided by end-point monitoring rather than strict adherence to a single formula (eg, Parkland) without real-time adjustments based on patient response.[53,54] The precise nature of those end points, however, is still controversial due to the complex series of variables which may impact the validity of said measurements—most notably urine output.

Table 3
A comparison of plasma products

	Fresh Frozen Plasma (FFP)	Reconstitued Lyophilized Plasma	Purified Protein Fraction (PPF)	5% Albumin
Albumin content (g/L)	35–50	30	36–45	50
Total protein content	60–80	50–52	43–50	50 (as albumina)
Sodium concentration	135–147	152	145–150	145
pH,Buffer	7.3–7.6 after thawinig, depending on duration of storage at 4 °C	8, no buffer	Sodium caprylate and acetyltryptophan or sodium carbonate	7.4, sodium bicarbonate or sodium hydroxide
Preservatives & anticoagulants	Citrate	None	None	None
Requires ABO compatibility with recipient	Yes	No	No	No

Comparison of the compostition of FFP, reconstituted lyophilized plasma, purified protein fraction.
From: Cartotto R, Callum J. A Review on the Use of Plasma During Acute Burn Resuscitation. J Burn Care Res. 2020;41(2):433 to 440. https://doi.org/10.1093/jbcr/irz184

New technologies in hemodynamic monitoring and tissue perfusion may add critical data to help finely tune resuscitative efforts and limit consequences of imperfect resuscitation. The next sections review traditional methods of monitoring and include new methods that could be used to guide resuscitative efforts in the future.

Traditional Methods

Noninvasive clinical measures

In the patient with a large burn, hourly urine output (UOP) monitored via indwelling Foley catheter has been the consensus parameter for decades that guides efforts. UOP indicates adequate perfusion of the kidney, a surrogate marker for overall intravascular volume status and CO. Optimal UOP has been suggested to be between 0.5 and 1 mL/kg for adults and 1 to 1.5 mL/kg for children, but this has never been verified experimentally.[27] A systematic review suggested UOP alone has similar outcomes on mortality when compared with more invasive hemodynamic monitoring.[55]

The use of UOP and vital signs alone to evaluate successful resuscitation has been called into question. A retrospective study comparing vital signs and UOP with oxygen consumption, oxygen delivery, and CO suggests that these traditional parameters alone do not sufficiently represent adequate resuscitation has occurred.[56] It is suggested that the particular impact of burns on renal function is somewhat disparate compared to other organs and therefore its use as a surrogate rather than a more centrally-oriented marker such as cardiovascular function may be insufficient.

Another quantitative end point that has been well-studied is lactic acid levels. Lactate is released from damaged or poorly perfused cells which causes metabolic acidosis upon intravascular accumulation. Elevated serum lactates or base deficits have been shown to correlate with mortality in critically ill patients and in burned patients. However, their use as guides for resuscitation is yet to be determined.[57] Following these markers over time can serve to confirm that resuscitation is occurring and that tissue perfusion is adequate. Normalization of base deficit after 24 hours has been associated with improved survival.[58] Conversely, elevated serum lactate after 48 hours is associated with increased mortality.[59] It is important to recognize that there are many possible etiologies for lactic acidosis that originate from different aspects of the total picture and require a detailed understanding of the individual patient and their clinical scenario to properly interpret.

Invasive monitoring

Vital signs obtained through noninvasive methods may be sufficient to supplement UOP. Often, especially in the case of burned extremities or with significant soft tissue edema, these data

Table 4
A comparison of vasopressors

Drug	Target	HR Inotropy	SVR	CO	BP	PVR	Main Users	Safe for PIV?
Inodilators								
Dobutamine 2–20 mck/kg/min	αβββ	↑↑↑	↓	↑↑↑	variable	↓	Cardiogenic shock	-
Milrinone 0.375–0.75 mcg/kg/min	cAMP	↑↑↑	↓↓	↑↑↑	variable	↓↓	Cardiogenic shock	-
Isoproterenol 2–10 mcg/min	ββββ	↑↑↑↑	↓	↑↑↑	variable	-	Bradycardia	Yes
Pure Vasopressors								
Vasopressin 0.01-0.06 U/min	VI & V2	↓	↑↑↑	↔/↓	↑↑↑	↓	Distributive shock, Pulmonary HTN	No
Phenylephrine 40–180 mcg/min	αααα	↓	↑↑↑	variable	↑↑↑	↑↑	Distributive shock, Pulmonary HTN	Yes
Inopressors								
Norepinephrine 0–40 mcg/min	αααβ	↑	↑↑↑	↔/↑	↑↑	↔	Shock	Yes < 24 hrs
Epinephrine 0–20 mcg/min	αβββ	↑↑↑	↑	↑↑↑	↑↑	-	Bradycardia, cardiogenic shock, sepsis, anaphylaxis	Yes
Dopamine (low) 1–4 mcg/kg/min	Dopa-R	↔	↓	↑	↓	-	Adjunct to other pressors	No
Dopamine (medium) 4–10 mcg/min	αβββD	↑	variable	↑↑	variable	-		
Dopamine (high) 10–20 mcg/kg/min	αααβD	↑↑	↑↑	↑	↑↑↑	↑		

Abbreviations: BP, blood pressure; CO, cardiac output; HR, heart rate; PIV, peripheral intravenous line; PVR, pulmonary vascular resistance; SVR, systemic vascular resistance.
Adapted from: Vasopressors. EMCrit Project. https://emcrit.org/ibcc/pressors/

may be imprecise and unreliable. Central line and arterial lines are more invasive methods that provide basic data about hemodynamics and volume status, including mean arterial pressure (MAP), central venous pressure (CVP), pulse pressure variation , and heart rate . However, CVP is more influenced by external or intraabdominal pressures (IAP) and may not be a true monitor of intravascular volume, particularly if bowel edema is further influencing IAP.[60]

In patients with pre-existing cardiac or renal disease, the pulmonary artery catheter (PAC) can be used to determine heart function and volume status. Hemodynamic data are obtained, such as pulmonary capillary wedge pressure (PCWP), pulmonary artery pressures, CO, cardiac index (CI), systemic vascular resistance (SVR), and oxygen consumption (Vo_2). The CO and CI are useful in determining cardiac sufficiency. PCWP and SVR are markers of volume status and shock. Vo_2 determines whether sufficient oxygen is delivered to tissues and whether these tissues are able to effectively extract the oxygen from the circulation. Taken together, these parameters create a larger picture of the cardiovascular system and end-organ perfusion.

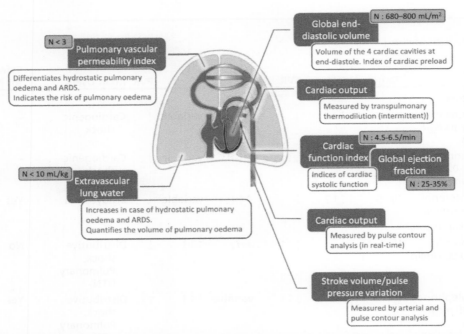

Fig. 3. Parameters measured by transpulmonary thermodilutionAlthough hypovolemia. (*From*: Monnet X, Teboul JL. Transpulmonary thermodilution: advantages and limits. Crit Care. 2017;21(1):147. https://doi.org/10.1186/s13054-017-1739-5)

In the burned patient, PCWP has been shown to be more reliable as a resuscitative marker than CVP.[61] Resuscitating to target CO has been linked to improved survival in burned patients.[62] Routine placement of the PAC and use of the previously mentioned variables correlates with improved survival.[63] However, there are potential complications to PAC placement, such as arrhythmias, blood clots, and damage or tearing of the pulmonary artery. Clearly, risks of placement of the PAC must be weighed against the benefits when guiding resuscitation. With advances in monitoring and imaging technologies, alternative techniques have become increasingly available to avoid the risk profile of PACs.

New monitoring adjuncts & alternatives

Newer technologies provide the opportunity to assess volume status in patients without the need for traditional invasive methods, like PACs, which provides new data with less risk to the patient. Transpulmonary thermodilution (TPTD), pulse contour analysis (PCA), and transesophageal echocardiography (TEE) are methods of obtaining hemodynamic parameters without the need for invasive maneuvers. Markers of tissue perfusion, such as subcutaneous gas tension or gastric tonometry, are also newly developing technologies that can add data to understanding burn resuscitation.

Requiring only a central line and an arterial line, TPTD can provide similar information as a PAC (**Fig. 3**) without the need for floating a balloon through the heart. Its use in burned patients has been studied and is reproducible and correlates well to data from the PAC.[64,65] These technologies have been studied in burned patients, but the evidence for their use as end points for resuscitation is still under investigation. A more recent study using TPTD found that it can be effectively used to identify those at increased risk for extravascular lung water in severely burned (>50% TBSA) patients using the intrathoracic blood volume index (ITBVI) which TPTD can calculate.[66] Implementation of TPTD to calculate such variables and identify ventilated patients at risk for pulmonary edema-related issues may help improve outcomes in patients with inhalation injury, but further studies are required. In addition, their utility is somewhat limited since their accuracy requires that a patient has no pre-existing cardiac disease and be paralyzed and on a mechanical ventilator.

Intrathoracic blood volume (ITBV) is a measurement obtained from TPTD that can be used to assess volume status and is a reflection of cardiac preload.[67] Other investigators have guided resuscitation based on ITBV end points. They found that ITBV targets were reached, whereas MAPS and UOP were below common end points. Thus, early resuscitation guided by ITBV targets seems safe and avoids unnecessary fluid input.[68]

However, there are competing data that show that resuscitating using ITBV results in using more fluid, more tissue edema, and shows no benefit to survival. Holm and colleagues have investigated ITBV as an end point of resuscitation in observational and prospective randomized studies.[69,70] Their research indicates that volumetric resuscitation to ITBV goals resulted in use of more fluid than predicted by the Baxter formula. With similar results, other researchers found that, in a comparative trial between resuscitation using the Parkland formula and traditional end points or resuscitation using ITBV, the group that received guided resuscitation by ITBV required more fluids and had subjectively more edema with no benefit to survival.[71]

PCAs (eg, LiDCO Plus, PiCCO Plus, and Flo-Trac) are another semi-invasive method of measuring CO and vital signs using thermodilution from a peripheral arterial catheter (**Fig. 4**). Their use in burned patients is contradictory. Reid and Jayamaha[55] first described the use in a case study in 2007 where they found it useful to adjust rates of fluid resuscitation based on measurements. In 2013, other authors measured the variation of stroke volume by PCA as it correlates with fluid administration.[72] These authors found that improvements in the pulse contour of patients with low CO were noted after rapid infusion of fluid, indicating a positive correlation to the volume given. Thus, they concluded that measuring stroke volume variation (SVV) by PCA might be a way to predict volume responsiveness in the early post-burn period. Moreover, a small 21-patient randomized controlled trial was conducted comparing goal-directed resuscitation in patients with PCA and SVV versus traditional end points, such as UOP and MAP.[73] Outcomes were similar but patients randomized to resuscitation based on the SVV received statistically significantly less crystalloid during the first 24 hours while having similar overall outcomes in terms of intensive care unit stay, duration of ventilation, and mortality.[74] Another study found that PCA metrics were similar to reference CO and SV measurements with a strong correlation to successful resuscitation albeit with a different trajectory than UOP-based monitoring.[75] In summary, PCA may be a useful adjunct to aid in resuscitation but, standing alone, may not be superior to traditional end points due to the theoretic and assumptive nature of many of the measurements as well as the impact of underlying factors on measurement validity.

Transthoracic echocardiography (TTE) and TEE allow direct visualization of the heart and intrathoracic vascular structures in real-time to facilitate dynamic functional interpretation. As with both PAC and PCA, echo allows assessment of cardiac parameters, such as CO and SVV, but gives additional information, such as cardiac valvular function, ejection fraction, and size and compressibility of the inferior vena cava. These data points can be monitored to evaluate real-time responsiveness to resuscitation efforts in a mixed quantitative and qualitative manner that other methods cannot provide. However, the quality of data, and subsequent adoption of this monitoring modality, has been limited due to their operator-dependent and assessor-dependent nature. Furthermore, placing a TEE probe is not without serious risk, such as esophageal perforation.

In 2003, researchers showed that patients are persistently hypovolemic according to TEE data, whereas other indicators of perfusion seem normal.[76] In 2008, researchers retrospectively studied a cohort of patients that had routinely received TEE during the acute phase of resuscitation. They concluded that TEE was valuable to assess real-time changes in hemodynamics but that the quality of data from TEE is not sufficient to replace traditional end points of resuscitation.[77] They suggested that TEE was useful as an adjunct in patients with pre-existing cardiac or renal function. Similarly, Bak and colleagues[78] recorded hemodynamic variables on 10 consecutive patients including with a TEE and a PAC but did not use those as end points to resuscitation, instead relying on UOP and MAP. They found that there was hypovolemia according to the TEE and PAC measurements during the first 12 hours of resuscitation. These measurements did not correlate with traditional measures of end organ perfusion, such as

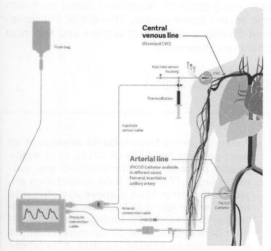

Fig. 4. Pulse contour analysis device (With permission from Pulsion Medical Systems SE, © 2023 Getinge.)

UOP, and corrected by 24 hours with no additional fluid resuscitation outside of what is recommended by the Parkland formula. They concluded that traditional methods are sufficient to guide resuscitation and that correcting for hypovolemia based on TEE measurements may lead to increased fluid administration without clinical benefit.

The most recent study looking at TEE utility in guiding burn resuscitation is from 2016 using a newer, smaller probe, less prone to esophageal complications and easy to navigate to the desired window. The study found that the TEE was able to guide fluid resuscitation and selection of inotropes to a specificity that broader clinical measures like UOP could not. The emphasis was that TEEs may provide a greater level of granularity than traditional methods, which can effectively direct resuscitation efforts in patients who have deviated from the standard course and have complicating cardiac factors requiring a higher level of assessment.[79]

Maintaining adequate end organ perfusion is the goal of burn resuscitation. Under-perfusion leads to conversion of partial thickness burns to full thickness. Devices that directly monitor the perfusion of the skin could therefore help guide resuscitation and improve salvage of deep partial-thickness burns. Subcutaneous tissue gas tension is measured with a fiberoptic device in the skin. Tissue pH, O_2, and CO_2 reflect perfusion of these tissues. Venkatesh and coworkers[80] studied subcutaneous gas tensions in a prospective series of 10 patients, which unexpectedly showed that perfusion in burned and unburned skin was similar during the resuscitation. Also, the research demonstrated deteriorating oxygenation, and therefore perfusion, of both burned and unburned tissue despite adequate resuscitation as assessed by traditional markers. This highlights a currently understudied and less frequently evaluated aspect of resuscitation compared to end-organ perfusion, which is assessment of capillary-level perfusion to the skin in burned and unburned areas.

A second small cohort study evaluated tissue gas tension and perfusion of a burned wound in response to resuscitation. In this series, the measured subcutaneous pH, a marker of poor wound perfusion, occurred before and predicted decreases in global markers of hypoperfusion, such as UOP, MAP, and lactates.[81]

Another rapidly advancing technology that will likely play an increasing role within burn assessment[82] and resuscitation[83] is laser doppler imaging. Currently, this technology is being developed for evaluating burn depth through real-time laser-based assessments of tissue perfusion. It has been used to predict burn depth and healing time, but with increased understanding of the technology,

it may be used to monitor dynamic changes in skin-level perfusion that can help reduce burn wound conversion and ensure adequate end-organ perfusion to the skin.[83]

Although using markers of tissue perfusion may lead to salvage of partial-thickness burns, resuscitating to these end points may lead to unnecessary administration of more fluid. A balance must be struck between maintaining perfusion of the skin against the multiple consequences of over-resuscitation, namely pulmonary edema and abdominal compartment syndrome. An area of expanding research and investment has occurred within computational and automated systems of tracking burn resuscitation. The capacity of computer-based systems to accurately calculate, track, and adjust ongoing resuscitative efforts is rapidly expanding.[84–86] Multiple software programs like Burn Navigator (©ARCOS Medical, Missouri City, TX, USA), BurnCase 3D (RISC Software GmbH) are being more widely utilized. As the ability of these programs to incorporate patient labs, wound healing progression, microbiology data, vitals, and other aspects of the global patient picture improves; their capacity to track, predict, and guide ongoing resuscitation will become even greater supplements to the burn provider's armamentarium. With the advent of AI technologies in recent years, the power of such programs will continue to grow as they will be able to learn from their decisions and past patients to enhance accuracy.

SUMMARY

Understanding the need and causes for fluid resuscitation after burn injury helps the clinician develop an effective plan to balance the competing goals of normalized tissue perfusion and limited tissue edema. Thoughtful, individualized treatment is the best answer and the most effective compromise.

CLINICS CARE POINTS

- Following initial trauma-based assessment of burn patients (ie, ABCs of ATLS), burn triage should proceed with standardized size estimates (ie, % TBSA) and fluid resuscitation implemented when TBSA is above 20%. Because of the central role that TBSA has in guiding interventions, especially during the acute 24-hour period, utilization of the correct method of burn size estimation is crucial as improper use of common methods can lead to over- and under-estimation by greater than 100%, which can have significant short- and long-term sequelae.

- During the initial 24-hour resuscitation window, capillary permeability is increased, causing burn-related systemic edema, but the exact timing of when this systemic effect resolves is contested, which has led to a variety of burn resuscitation algorithms with and without the use of colloid during that time. Consideration of unique patient factors and the degree of response to ongoing resuscitation efforts should guide implementation of colloids during this window. Those who use colloid in the first 24 hours often advocate for waiting at least 8-12 hours before their implementation based on existing studies.

- While the rBaux Score (%TBSA + age + 17 [if INHI present]) is a useful tool to guide discussions on burn morbidity with families, it should be used with caution as a direct correlate for mortality predictions due to the high predictive variability seen across the literature. As burn care becomes more advanced and patients are treated at increasingly specialized centers, the reliability of predictive scores like rBaux and others will waver and require further adjustment to modern practice.

- While urine output is the most common parameter used to titrate acute burn resuscitation to prevent over- and under-resuscitation, factors such as multisystem organ failure with renal involvement or other pathologies that impair renal perfusion unrelated to intravascular volume status may significantly impact the reliability of urine output for monitoring volume status. Useful adjuncts such as bedside ultrasound of cardiac function and inferior vena cava collapsibility, straight-leg raise test, and newer non-invasive technologies may all be added to the ongoing assessment of critically ill patients with renal function impairment to more thoroughly assess the adequacy of ongoing fluid resuscitation.

DISCLOSURE

The authors have no relevant financial or conflict of interest disclosures to make as it relates to the topic of this article.

REFERENCES

1. Cartotto R, Callum J. A review of the use of human albumin in burn patients. J Burn Care Res 2012; 33(6):702–17.

2. Bingham HG. Role of thermal injury-induced hypoproteinemia on fluid flux and protein permeability in burned and non-burned tissue. Plast Reconstr Surg 1963 1984;74(6):862.

3. Szczesny B, Brunyánszki A, Ahmad A, et al. Time-dependent and organ-specific changes in mitochondrial function, mitochondrial DNA integrity, oxidative stress and mononuclear cell infiltration in a mouse model of burn injury. PLoS One 2015; 10(12):e0143730.

4. Kao CC, Garner WL. Acute burns. Plast Reconstr Surg 1963 2000;105(7):2482–92.

5. Warden GD. Fluid resuscitation and early management. In: Total burn care. 4th Edition. Elsevier - Health Sciences Division; 2012. p. 115–24.e3. https://doi.org/10.1016/B978-1-4377-2786-9.00009-6.

6. Modi S, Rashid M, Malik A, et al. Study of complement activation, C3 and interleukin-6 levels in burn patients and their role as prognostic markers. Indian J Med Microbiol 2014;32(2):137–42.

7. Matsuura H, Matsumoto H, Osuka A, et al. Clinical importance of a cytokine network in major burns. Shock 2019;51(2):185–93.

8. Tricklebank S. Modern trends in fluid therapy for burns. Burns 2009;35(6):757–67.

9. Wurzer P, Culnan D, Cancio LC, et al. 8 - pathophysiology of burn shock and burn edema. In: Herndon DN, editor. Total burn care. 5th Edition. Elsevier; 2018. p. 66–76.e3. https://doi.org/10.1016/B978-0-323-47661-4.00008-3.

10. Tejiram S, Tranchina SP, Travis TE, et al. The first 24 hours: burn shock resuscitation and early complications. Surg Clin North Am 2023;103(3):403–13.

11. Moore EE, Moore HB, Kornblith LZ, et al. Trauma-induced coagulopathy. Nat Rev Dis Primer 2021; 7(1):1–23.

12. Hilton JG, Marullo DS. Effects of thermal trauma on cardiac force of contraction. Burns 1986;12(3):167–71.

13. Horton JW, Maass DL, White DJ, et al. Effects of burn serum on myocardial inflammation and function. Shock Augusta Ga 2004;22(5):438–45.

14. Holm C, Hörbrand F, Henckel von Donnersmarck G, et al. Acute renal failure in severely burned patients. Burns 1999;25(2):171–8.

15. Chrysopoulo MT, Jeschke MG, Dziewulski P, et al. Acute renal dysfunction in severely burned adults. J Trauma Inj Infect Crit Care 1999;46(1):141–4.

16. Garner WL, Magee W. Acute burn injury. Clin Plast Surg 2005;32(2):187–93.

17. Jeschke MG, van Baar ME, Choudhry MA, et al. Burn injury. Nat Rev Dis Primer 2020;6(1):11.

18. Oda J, Yamashita K, Inoue T, et al. Resuscitation fluid volume and abdominal compartment syndrome in patients with major burns. Burns 2006;32(2): 151–4.

19. Rizzo JA, Liu NT, Coates EC, et al. The battle of the titans-comparing resuscitation between five major burn centers using the burn navigator. J Burn Care Res 2023;44(2):446–51.

20. Freiburg C, Igneri P, Sartorelli K, et al. Effects of differences in percent total body surface area

estimation on fluid resuscitation of transferred burn patients. J Burn Care Res 2007;28(1):42–8.

21. Saffle JR. The phenomenon of "fluid creep" in acute burn resuscitation. J Burn Care Res 2007;28(3):382–95.

22. Cancio LC, Chávez S, Alvarado-Ortega M, et al. Predicting increased fluid requirements during the resuscitation of thermally injured patients. J Trauma 2004;56(2):404–14.

23. Ivy ME, Atweh NA, Palmer J, et al. Intra-abdominal hypertension and abdominal compartment syndrome in burn patients. J Trauma Inj Infect Crit Care 2000;49(3):387–91.

24. Blumetti J, Hunt JL, Arnoldo BD, et al. The Parkland formula under fire: is the criticism justified? J Burn Care Res 2008;29(1):180–6.

25. Grunwald TB, Garner WL. Acute burns. Plast Reconstr Surg 2008;121(5):311e–9e.

26. American Burn Association. Advanced Burn Life Support Handbook.; 2018.

27. Pham TN, Cancio LC, Gibran NS, et al. American burn association practice guidelines burn shock resuscitation. J Burn Care Res 2008;29(1):257–66.

28. Singh S, Kerndt CC, Davis D. Ringer's lactate. In: StatPearls. StatPearls Publishing; 2023. http://www.ncbi.nlm.nih.gov/books/NBK500033/. Accessed July 30, 2023.

29. Monafo WW. The treatment of burn shock by the intravenous and oral administration of hypertonic lactated saline solution. J Trauma 1970;10(7):575–86.

30. Dulhunty JM, Boots RJ, Rudd MJ, et al. Increased fluid resuscitation can lead to adverse outcomes in major-burn injured patients, but low mortality is achievable. Burns 2008;34(8):1090–7.

31. Huang PP, Stucky FS, Dimick AR, et al. Hypertonic sodium resuscitation is associated with renal failure and death. Ann Surg 1995;221(5):543–57.

32. Monafo WW. Initial management of burns. N Engl J Med 1996;335(21):1581–6.

33. Cochran A, Morris SE, Edelman LS, et al. Burn patient characteristics and outcomes following resuscitation with albumin. Burns 2007;33(1):25–30.

34. Goodwin CW, Dorethy J, Lam V, et al. Randomized trial of efficacy of crystalloid and colloid resuscitation on hemodynamic response and lung water following thermal injury. Ann Surg 1983;197(5):520–31.

35. Béchir M, Puhan MA, Fasshauer M, et al. Early fluid resuscitation with hydroxyethyl starch 130/0.4 (6%) in severe burn injury: a randomized, controlled, double-blind clinical trial. Crit Care Lond Engl 2013;17(6):R299.

36. Perel P, Roberts I, Ker K. Colloids versus crystalloids for fluid resuscitation in critically ill patients. Cochrane Database Syst Rev 2013;2:CD000567.

37. Vlachou E, Gosling P, Moiemen NS. Microalbuminuria: a marker of endothelial dysfunction in thermal injury. Burns 2006;32(8):1009–16.

38. Wisner DH, Street D, Demling R. Effect of colloid versus crystalloid resuscitation on soft tissue edema formation. Curr Surg 1983;40(1):32–5.

39. Du GB, Slater H, Goldfarb IW. Influences of different resuscitation regimens on acute early weight gain in extensively burned patients. Burns 1991;17(2):147–50.

40. Navickis RJ, Greenhalgh DG, Wilkes MM. Albumin in burn shock resuscitation: a meta-analysis of controlled clinical studies. J Burn Care Res 2016;37(3):e268–78.

41. Greenhalgh DG, Cartotto R, Taylor SL, et al. Burn resuscitation practices in north America: results of the acute burn resuscitation multicenter prospective trial (ABRUPT). Ann Surg 2023;277(3):512–9.

42. O'Mara MS, Slater H, Goldfarb IW, et al. A prospective, randomized evaluation of intra-abdominal pressures with crystalloid and colloid resuscitation in burn patients. J Trauma 2005;58(5):1011–8.

43. Selahattin V, Yasti CA, Mete D. Comparison of albumin and fresh frozen plasma as colloid therapy in patients with major burns. Cureus 2023;15(1). https://doi.org/10.7759/cureus.33485.

44. Kahn S, Boyde B, ONeill K, et al. 58 Achieving < 2cc/kg/%TBSA - a restrictive adjusted ideal body weight resuscitation formula with fresh frozen plasma. J Burn Care Res 2023;44(Supplement_2):S26–7.

45. Wiktor AJ, Carmichael H, Weber EB, et al. 85 safety and efficacy of early fresh frozen plasma administration in burn resuscitation. J Burn Care Res 2020;41(Supplement_1):S55–6.

46. Bunn F, Trivedi D, Bunn F. Colloid solutions for fluid resuscitation. Cochrane Database Syst Rev 2012;2012(11):CD001319.

47. Cartotto R, Callum J. A review on the use of plasma during acute burn resuscitation. J Burn Care Res 2020;41(2):433–40.

48. Matsuda T, Tanaka H, Shimazaki S, et al. High-dose vitamin C therapy for extensive deep dermal burns. Burns 1992;18(2):127–31.

49. Tanaka H, Matsuda T, Miyagantani Y, et al. Reduction of resuscitation fluid volumes in severely burned patients using ascorbic acid administration: a randomized, prospective study. Arch Surg 2000;135(3):326–31.

50. Kahn SA, Beers RJ, Lentz CW. Resuscitation after severe burn injury using high-dose ascorbic acid: a retrospective review. J Burn Care Res 2011;32(1):110–7.

51. Siddiqi M, Evans T, Guiab K, et al. Vitamin C in the management of burn patients: a systematic review of the risks and benefits. Am Surg 2022;88(4):752–7.

52. Buehner M, Pamplin J, Studer L, et al. Oxalate nephropathy after continuous infusion of high-dose vitamin c as an adjunct to burn resuscitation. J Burn Care Res 2016;37(4):e374–9.

53. Greenhalgh DG. Burn resuscitation. J Burn Care Res 2007;28(4):555–65.

54. Arlati S, Storti E, Pradella V, et al. Decreased fluid volume to reduce organ damage: a new approach to burn shock resuscitation? a preliminary study. Resuscitation 2007;72(3):371–8.

55. Paratz JD, Stockton K, Paratz ED, et al. Burn resuscitation—hourly urine output versus alternative endpoints: a systematic review. Shock Augusta Ga 2014;42(4):295–306.

56. Dries DJ, Waxman K. Adequate resuscitation of burn patients may not be measured by urine output and vital signs. Crit Care Med 1991;19(3):327–9.

57. Cartotto R. Fluid resuscitation of the thermally injured patient. Clin Plast Surg 2009;36(4):569–81.

58. Andel D, Kamolz LP, Roka J, et al. Base deficit and lactate: early predictors of morbidity and mortality in patients with burns. Burns 2007;33(8):973–8.

59. Cochran A, Edelman LS, Saffle JR, et al. The relationship of serum lactate and base deficit in burn patients to mortality. J Burn Care Res 2007;28(2): 231–40.

60. Küntscher MV, Germann G, Hartmann B. Correlations between cardiac output, stroke volume, central venous pressure, intra-abdominal pressure and total circulating blood volume in resuscitation of major burns. Resuscitation 2006;70(1):37–43.

61. Aikawa N, Martyn J, Burke JF. Pulmonary artery catheterization and thermodilution cardiac output determination in the management of critically burned patients. Am J Surg 1978;135(6):811–7.

62. Agarwal N, Petro J, Salisbury RE. Physiologic profile monitoring in burned patients. J Trauma 1983;23(7): 577–83.

63. Schiller WR, Bay RC. Hemodynamic and oxygen transport monitoring in management of burns. New Horiz Baltim Md 1996;4(4):475–82.

64. Küntscher MV, Blome-Eberwein S, Pelzer M, et al. Transcardiopulmonary vs pulmonary arterial thermodilution methods for hemodynamic monitoring of burned patients. J Burn Care Rehabil 2002;23(1): 21–6.

65. Holm C, Mayr M, Hörbrand F, et al. Reproducibility of transpulmonary thermodilution measurements in patients with burn shock and hypothermia. J Burn Care Rehabil 2005;26(3):260–5.

66. Wang W, Yu X, Zuo F, et al. Risk factors and the associated limit values for abnormal elevation of extravascular lung water in severely burned adults. Burns 2019;45(4):849–59.

67. Wiesenack C, Prasser C, Keyl C, et al. Assessment of intrathoracic blood volume as an indicator of cardiac preload: single transpulmonary thermodilution technique versus assessment of pressure preload parameters derived from a pulmonary artery catheter. J Cardiothorac Vasc Anesth 2001;15(5): 584–8.

68. Sánchez M, García-de-Lorenzo A, Herrero E, et al. A protocol for resuscitation of severe burn patients guided by transpulmonary thermodilution and lactate levels: a 3-year prospective cohort study. Crit Care Lond Engl 2013;17(4):R176.

69. Holm C, Melcer B, Hörbrand F, et al. Intrathoracic blood volume as an end point in resuscitation of the severely burned: an observational study of 24 patients. J Trauma 2000;48(4):728–34.

70. Holm C, Mayr M, Tegeler J, et al. A clinical randomized study on the effects of invasive monitoring on burn shock resuscitation. Burns 2004;30(8):798–807.

71. Aboelatta Y, Abdelsalam A. Volume overload of fluid resuscitation in acutely burned patients using transpulmonary thermodilution technique. J Burn Care Res 2013;34(3):349–54.

72. Lavrentieva A, Kontakiotis T, Kaimakamis E, et al. Evaluation of arterial waveform derived variables for an assessment of volume resuscitation in mechanically ventilated burn patients. Burns 2013; 39(2):249–54.

73. Reid RD, Jayamaha J. The use of a cardiac output monitor to guide the initial fluid resuscitation in a patient with burns. Emerg Med J EMJ 2007;24(5):e32.

74. Tokarik M, Sjöberg F, Balik M, et al. Fluid therapy LiDCO controlled trial-optimization of volume resuscitation of extensively burned patients through noninvasive continuous real-time hemodynamic monitoring LiDCO. J Burn Care Res 2013;34(5): 537–42.

75. ArabiDarrehDor G, Kao YM, Oliver MA, et al. The potential of arterial pulse wave analysis in burn resuscitation: a pilot in vivo study. J Burn Care Res 2023;44(3):599–609.

76. Papp A, Uusaro A, Parviainen I, et al. Myocardial function and haemodynamics in extensive burn trauma: evaluation by clinical signs, invasive monitoring, echocardiography and cytokine concentrations. A prospective clinical study. Acta Anaesthesiol Scand 2003;47(10):1257–63.

77. Wang GY, Ma B, Tang HT, et al. Esophageal echo-Doppler monitoring in burn shock resuscitation: are hemodynamic variables the critical standard guiding fluid therapy? J Trauma 2008;65(6):1396–401.

78. Bak Z, Sjöberg F, Eriksson O, et al. Hemodynamic changes during resuscitation after burns using the parkland formula. J Trauma 2009;66(2):329–36.

79. Held JM, Litt J, Kennedy JD, et al. Surgeon-performed hemodynamic transesophageal echocardiography in the burn intensive care unit. J Burn Care Res 2016; 37(1):e63–8.

80. Venkatesh B, Meacher R, Muller MJ, et al. Monitoring tissue oxygenation during resuscitation of major burns. J Trauma Inj Infect Crit Care 2001;50(3): 485–94.

81. Jeng JC, Jaskille AD, Lunsford PM, et al. Improved markers for burn wound perfusion in the severely

burned patient: the role for tissue and gastric PCO2. J Burn Care Res 2008;29(1):49–55.

82. Hoeksema H, Van de Sijpe K, Tondu T, et al. Accuracy of early burn depth assessment by laser Doppler imaging on different days post burn. Burns 2009;35(1):36–45.

83. Shahid S, Duarte MC, Zhang J, et al. Laser Doppler imaging – the role of poor burn perfusion in predicting healing time and guiding operative management. Burns 2023;49(1):129–36.

84. Salinas J, Chung KK, Mann EA, et al. Computerized decision support system improves fluid resuscitation following severe burns: an original study. Crit Care Med 2011;39(9):2031–8.

85. Monnet X, Teboul JL. Transpulmonary thermodilution: advantages and limits. Crit Care 2017;21(1):147.

86. Bijl RC, Valensise H, Novelli GP, et al. Methods and considerations concerning cardiac output measurement in pregnant women: recommendations of the International Working Group on Maternal Hemodynamics. Ultrasound Obstet Gynecol 2019;54(1):35–50.

Inhalation Injury, Respiratory Failure, and Ventilator Support in Acute Burn Care

Sai R. Velamuri, MD[a],*, Yasmin Ali, MD, MPH[b], Julio Lanfranco, MD, MPH[c],
Pooja Gupta, MD[d], David M. Hill, PharmD, BCPS, BCCCP, FCCM[e]

KEYWORDS

- Burns • Inhalation injury • Acute lung injury • Ventilators • Mechanical • Extracorporeal circulation
- Therapeutics

KEY POINTS

- Management of inhalation injuries is complex and significantly increases the risk of morbidity and mortality.
- There remains a paucity of quality evidence to guide treatment.
- There is no universally accepted ventilation mode and setting should be customized according to patient compliance, airway resistance, and work of breathing.

INTRODUCTION/EPIDEMIOLOGY

The management of a large burn can prove to be extremely challenging. When this is compounded by the presence of smoke inhalation, the care gets even more complex with a significant increase in both morbidity and mortality.[1,2] The Cocoanut Grove fire was a nightclub fire which took place in Boston, Massachusetts, on November 28, 1942, resulting in the deaths of 492 people.[3,4] The majority who perished on the scene suffered from smoke inhalation.

Inhalation injury is defined as the aspiration and/or inhalation of superheated gasses, steam, hot liquids, or noxious products of incomplete combustion (found in smoke).[5] The severity of the injury is related to the temperature, composition, and length of exposure to the inhaled agent. The incidence is around 2% to 14% of patients admitted to burn centers. Inhalation injury can occur with or without a skin burn. A significant number of fire-related deaths are not due to the skin burn, but to the toxic effects of the by-products of combustion (airborne particles). Burns that are associated with carbon monoxide (CO) and/or hydrogen cyanide (CN) poisoning, hypoxia, and upper airway edema can pose serious challenges during the early clinical course of a patient with inhalation injury. Individuals of all age (pediatric/adults and seniors) are at a higher risk of death when their thermal injury is complicated by smoke inhalation.[6] Inhalation injury greatly increases the incidence of respiratory failure, acute respiratory distress syndrome (ARDS), and death.

[a] Department of Surgery, College of Medicine, University of Tennessee, Health Science Center, Memphis, TN 38103, USA; [b] Department of Surgery, College of Medicine, University of Tennessee Health Science Center, 910 Madison Avenue, 2nd floor Suite 217, Memphis, TN 38103, USA; [c] Division of Pulmonary and Critical Care, University of Tennessee Health Science Center, 965 Court Avenue Room H316B, Memphis, TN 38103, USA; [d] Pulmonary and Critical Care, University of Tennessee Health Science Center, 965 court avenue, Room H316B, Memphis, TN 38103, USA; [e] Department of Pharmacy, Regional One Health, University of Tennessee, 80 madison avenue, Memphis TN 38103, USA
* Corresponding author. 890 Madison Avenue, TG 032, Memphis, TN 38103.
E-mail address: svelamur@uthsc.edu

Clin Plastic Surg 51 (2024) 221–232
https://doi.org/10.1016/j.cps.2023.11.001
0094-1298/24/© 2023 Elsevier Inc. All rights reserved.

PATHOPHYSIOLOGY

Upper airway injuries are usually a result of thermal injuries and involve the mouth, oropharynx, and larynx.[5] In rare cases, such as steam inhalation in an enclosed space, heat can cause subglottic injury.[5,7] Lower airway injuries tend to be caused by chemical injuries or particulate matter from smoke and involve the trachea, bronchi, and alveoli.[5]

Thermal injury to the airway causes denaturation of proteins, which activates the complement cascade and the release of histamine.[8] It also releases free radicals, which combine with nitric oxide in the endothelium of the airway and cause airway edema by increasing the microvascular pressure and tissue permeability.[8] The continued presence of pro-inflammatory cytokines and free radicals leads to worsening airway edema, contributing to increased resuscitation requirements during acute burn resuscitation.[8]

Generally, the upper airway protects the lower airway from heat, so lower airway inhalation injury is usually caused by the chemicals present in smoke, which cause a pro-inflammatory response due to their caustic nature.[8] The presence of chemicals in the airways causes increased bronchial blood flow, which leads to increased permeability and destruction of the bronchial epithelium as well as bronchospasm.[7,8] Bronchial blood flow is increased 10-fold, secondary to local cellular damage, and loss of hypoxic pulmonary vasoconstriction.[8,9] Initially, the goblet cells produce copious secretions, which eventually harden and become casts, causing airway obstruction.[8] The coagulation cascade is also initiated during an injury secondary to smoke inhalation.[10] This occurs due to a combination of coagulation factors from plasma exuded following vascular injury, tissue factor present in pulmonary endothelial cells, and alveolar macrophages, which results in fibrin deposits in the alveolar space.[10] The combination of loss of hypoxic pulmonary vasoconstriction, increased blood flow to injured lung parenchyma, decreased ventilation of collapsed lung segments, decreased pulmonary compliance, increased pulmonary resistance, and edema contributes to ventilation-perfusion mismatch and profound hypoxemia.[8,9]

DIAGNOSIS

Patients with acute burn injury are evaluated initially using the Advanced Burn Life Support protocol. After the primary survey using ABCDE (Airway, Breathing, Circulation, Disability, Exposure), the secondary survey calculates the percentage total burn surface area (TBSA) involved. A proper history

---

Box 1
Considerations to aid diagnosis of inhalation injury

History
- Reported mechanism of burn
- Potential and duration of exposure to flame, smoke, or chemicals
- Exposure in an enclosed space
- Loss of consciousness or disability
- Headache, delirium, hallucinations, or comatose
- Burning sensation in the nose or throat
- Cough with increased sputum production
- Stridor or odynophagia after smoke exposure
- Wheezing or dyspnea with rhonchi

Examination
- Facial burns, singed eyebrows, facial, or nasal hair
- Soot or carbonaceous material on the face, airway, or sputum
- Signs of upper airway obstruction (eg, hoarseness, retraction, stridor, drooling, dysphagia)
- Suspicion of lower airway disease (eg, tachypnea, decreased breath sounds, wheezing, rales, rhonchi, or use of accessory respiratory muscles)

Laboratory test
- Complete blood count
- Basic metabolic panel (blood urea nitrogen, creatinine, electrolytes)
- Lactate
- Toxicology screen
- Arterial blood gas
- Carboxylated hemoglobin and methemoglobin
- Cyanide concentration

Imaging
- Chest radiograph
- Bronchoscopy
- Computed tomography of the chest

---

and examination are done to determine the likelihood of inhalation injury (**Box 1**).

Considering the presence of inhalation injury is an independent predictor of mortality, and it is crucial to have a high index of suspicion.[9] Fiberoptic bronchoscopy, radionuclide imaging with [133]Xenon, computed tomography (CT), elevated carboxyhemoglobin (COHb), and pulmonary function testing (PFT) have all been considered for diagnosing inhalation injury. Bronchoscopy is now considered the gold standard for diagnosing inhalation injury.[11] Testing with xenon-133 or PFT is not always available or acutely practical. Hassan and colleagues demonstrated the arterial partial pressure of oxygen to the fraction of inspired oxygen ratio (P/F) as a predictor of survival once the initial burn resuscitation has been completed.[12] However, the P/F is easily affected by the mode of ventilation as well as resuscitation volumes. Patients with inhalation injury may present with a normal chest radiograph and arterial blood gas. Oh and colleagues found that the radiologist's score added to bronchoscopy findings could enhance prognostication of a composite endpoint of pneumonia, acute lung injury/ARDS, and death.[13] Yamamura and colleagues showed that CT findings of greater than 3.0 mm bronchial wall thickness 2 cm distal to the carina had a statistically significant correlation with development of pneumonia, number of days on ventilator, and intensive care unit (ICU) length of stay.[14] CT findings could be used complementary to bronchoscopy findings.

BRONCHOSCOPY

Bronchoscopic findings can be important in managing patients and can also have therapeutic effects.[15,16] Hassan and colleagues showed TBSA, age, and bronchoscopic findings had a positive correlation with mortality.[12] Flexible bronchoscopy is unable to evaluate damage in the distal airways leading to sometimes discordance in bronchoscopy findings and overall mortality. Patients with inhalation injury are at high risk of ventilator-associated pneumonia, increasing mortality risk upward of 60%.[17] It is a common practice to obtain bronchoalveolar lavage at the time of bronchoscopy.

Bronchoscopy has been used for suctioning out inspissated secretions, casts, and foreign bodies, which may be causing airway obstruction. The most commonly used grading system is the Abbreviated Injury Scale, which takes into account absence or presence of carbonaceous deposits, erythema, edema, bronchorrhea, or obstruction.[18]

The role of repeated bronchoscopies remains controversial, and literature has only retrospective studies or case reports. A retrospective review showed a decreased duration of mechanical ventilation (MV), shorter length of ICU stay, and hospital stay for patients who underwent repeated bronchoscopies. There was also a trend toward mortality benefit favoring repeated bronchoscopies.[19] It has become a common practice to perform repeated daily bronchoscopies in patients with initial grade 2 or higher degree of inhalation injury.

INTUBATION

The focus of airway management during the first 24 hours is to maintain airway patency with adequate oxygenation and ventilation. Inhalation injury frequently increases respiratory secretions and may generate a large amount of carbonaceous debris in the patient's respiratory tract. Frequent and adequate suctioning is necessary to prevent occlusion of the airway and endotracheal tube (ETT). Orotracheal intubation using a cuffed ETT is preferred. In adults, if possible, the ETT should be of sufficient size to permit adequate pulmonary toilet and diagnostic and therapeutic bronchoscopy following transfer to the burn center.[20] In children, cuffed ETTs are also preferred using an age-appropriate size. In instances where non-burn trauma mandates cervical spine protection (eg, motor vehicle collisions and falls), cervical spine stabilization is critical during intubation. In impending airway obstruction, clearance of the cervical spine should be postponed.

Indications for early intubation:

- Signs of airway obstruction: hoarseness, stridor, accessory respiratory muscle use, sternal retraction
- Extent of the burn (TBSA burn greater than 40%–50%)
- Extensive and deep facial burns
- Burns inside the mouth
- Significant edema or risk for edema
- Difficulty swallowing
- Signs of respiratory compromise (ie, inability to clear secretions, respiratory fatigue, poor oxygenation, or ventilation)
- Decreased level of consciousness where airway protective reflexes are impaired
- Anticipated patient transfer of large burn with airway issue without qualified personnel to intubate in route

The timing of intubation in burn patients with inhalation injury is crucial. Esnault and colleagues showed patients with face and neck burns who were intubated at the burn center had a five times higher chance of encountering a difficult intubation as compared with prehospital intubation by Emergency Medical Services (EMS).[21] With increasing facial swelling and edema, there may be distortion of the normal upper airway anatomy making intubation difficult.

Although it is important to intubate patients in a timely manner, it is equally essential to avoid unnecessary intubations. A recent retrospective analysis showed that one-third of the intubated patients were extubated within 24 hours and more patients intubated at a non-burn center had early extubation compared with patients intubated at a burn center or by EMS (42% vs 20%).[22] Almost 80% of patients extubated early did not have any evidence of inhalation injury. This study underlines the importance of quickly getting patient to an experienced burn center to correctly identifying patients with inhalation injury.

EARLY TRACHEOSTOMY

Tracheostomy is a commonly performed procedure in critical care and helps in ventilation weaning, reducing amount of sedation required, decreasing ICU delirium, and improving bronchial hygiene with a secure airway. The literature however is controversial when it comes to using tracheostomy for burn patients with inhalation injuries. Laryngotracheal stenosis may occur in up to 24% of patients with inhalation injury.[23] Aggarwal and colleagues did not show any mortality difference in burn patients who underwent tracheostomy versus those who did not.[24] Although evidence does not support prophylactic tracheostomies, a survival benefit was seen with tracheostomy in patients with 60% TBSA burns.[24] Tracheostomy is not associated with increased pneumonia; however, persistent tracheostomy is a commonly reported complication.

Tsuchiya and colleagues showed that there is no mortality difference between early (mean day 4) versus late (mean 2 weeks) tracheostomies in burn patients.[25] Early tracheostomy however has been associated with improvement of the P/F, fewer days on MV, shorter hospital length of stay, and earlier first day of active exercises.[26,27] There is a 16 times increased risk of dysphagia in burn patients with inhalation injury compared with patients without inhalation injury.[28] Smailes and colleagues showed that this risk of dysphagia increased if tracheostomy was performed more than 7 days after oral intubation and early tracheostomy could potentially decrease this risk of developing dysphagia.[29] Stefan and colleagues published a normogram to predict the need for tracheostomy in which age, TBSA, and inhalation injury were significant factors. Further studies will be needed to validate the utility of the normogram in clinical practice.[30]

HIGH VERSUS LOW TIDAL VOLUME VENTILATION

Low tidal volume ventilation has consistently been validated for the treatment of ARDS in adults.[31] This MV strategy has shown to improve morbidity and mortality from ARDS.[32] Lung-protective ventilation is based on the principle of limited tidal

volumes (6–8 mL/Kg of ideal body weight and plateau pressures of <30 cm H_2O). However, the ARDSNET trial excluded burn patients with greater than 30% TBSA.

Given the unique characteristics of burn patients, such as airway obstruction from fibrin casts and decreased chest compliance, low tidal column ventilation can be challenging. In contrast, a single retrospective study on pediatric patients suffering from inhalation injury found that high tidal volume ventilation (15 ± 3 mL/kg) significantly decreased ventilator days and the incidence of both atelectasis and ARDS.[20] Although optimal tidal volume remains undefined, most experts recommend limiting tidal volumes to the lowest level tolerated by the patient's compliance, airway resistance, and work of breathing.[33]

MODES OF MECHANICAL VENTILATION

Ventilator management of patients with inhalation injury might deviate from conventional practices given their unique physiology. Currently, there is no single ventilator mode that prevails, and this is due to a paucity of clinical trials. Larger randomized trials are needed to elucidate what is the best mode of MV for patients with inhalation injuries. Chung and colleagues found that conventional modes, particularly pressure support ventilation and volume-assist control modes, were the most used modes in North America.[33] However, unconventional modes are also being used as discussed.[9] If a conventional mode is to be used, providers should aim to limit the tidal volume to the lowest level tolerated by the patient's compliance and airway resistance.

Airway Pressure Release Ventilation

Airway pressure release ventilation (APRV) is an inverse ratio, pressure-controlled mode of ventilation that allows for spontaneous breaths.[8] APRV has not been shown to improve survival. One trial conducted in China, on patients with ARDS, found that APRV use was associated with shorter durations of both MV and ICU stay.[34] Batchinsky and colleagues found no survival benefit of APRV use versus conventional therapy in patients with inhalation injury and respiratory failure.[35]

High-Frequency Percussive Ventilation

Cioffi and colleagues first described high-frequency percussive ventilation (HFPV) in 1989 as a mean of ventilatory support, assisting with clearance of secretions, as well as decreasing barotrauma and pneumonia.[36] HFPV delivers very small, high-frequency tidal breaths that lower airway pressures as well as produce intrabronchial percussion and airway turbulence. This action helps mobilization and clearance of secretions and plugs.[7]

The use of prophylactic HFPV in patients with inhalation injury has demonstrated benefits in mortality, incidence of pulmonary infection, and barotrauma; however, it is important to mention that this study on 54 patients between 1987 and 1990 was compared with a historic cohort.[37] In a single-center prospective, randomized, controlled clinical trial, comparing HFPV with low tidal volume ventilation in patients admitted to a burn intensive care unit with respiratory failure (approximately 35% had inhalation injury), the researchers found no difference in ventilator-free days or mortality.[38]

High-Frequency Oscillatory Ventilation

High-frequency oscillatory ventilation delivers very small tidal volumes at high frequency to maximize lung recruitment with sustained mean airway pressure.[39] Given the pathophysiology of inhalation injury and bronchial obstructive changes, this mode is unlikely to be effective. Cartotto and colleagues compared patients with ARDS secondary to inhalation injury versus ARDS from burns without inhalation injuries and found that the former group had worsening hypoxia and hypercapnia.[40] This ventilation strategy has also failed to prove any benefit on ARDS patients without inhalation injury in two large randomized controlled trials.[41,42]

Extracorporeal Membrane Oxygenation

Extracorporeal membrane oxygenation (ECMO) is usually seen as a rescue strategy when every other measure to improve oxygenation has failed. Data on burn patients are extremely scarce. A meta-analysis published in 2013 showed no improvement in survival for burn patients suffering from acute hypoxemic respiratory failure.[43] A recent registry showed that the mortality of burn patients (inhalation injury 26.7%) receiving ECMO was comparable that for non-burn ECMO patients.[44]

COMPLICATIONS
Pulmonary Edema

Pulmonary edema is the excessive accumulation of fluid in the lung parenchyma. Non-cardiogenic pulmonary edema is caused by increase in capillary permeability and changes in the pulmonary gradient within the pulmonary capillaries.[45] Pulmonary edema occurs in the presence of inhalation injury but may be worsened during acute burn resuscitation. Those with inhalation injuries commonly require higher than calculated resuscitation, which increases the risk for pulmonary edema and other complications associated with over resuscitation. Fluid creep is a phenomenon, described by Pruitt, in which more fluid is given than is calculated using the standard formulas.[46] This results in abdominal and extremity compartment syndrome, pulmonary and cerebral edema, ARDS, and multiple organ failure, thereby increasing morbidity and mortality in burn patients.[46]

Acute Respiratory Distress Syndrome
Epidemiology
ARDS was originally described by Ashbaugh and colleagues.[47] Later, in 2012, the ARDS task force introduced the Berlin definition; this criterion specifies risk factors, timing of onset, and replaces the previous acute lung injury category by identifying three levels of ARDS severity. The levels of ARDS severity are based on P/F.[48]

Patients suffering from either cutaneous burns or inhalation injury are at an increased risk of developing ARDS. Belenkiy and colleagues found that 33% of mechanically ventilated burn patients developed ARDS and these patients had a mortality rate of 33%.[49] Lam and colleagues found that patients with inhalation injury developed ARDS sooner and were more hypoxic when compared with burn patients without inhalation injury.[50]

Protective ventilation
Burn patients with ARDS have historically been excluded from clinical trials. Based on the ARDS-net findings on non-burn patients, low tidal volume ventilation (6–8 mL/Kg of ideal body weight and plateau pressures of <30 cm H_2O) has consistently shown decreased mortality as well as decreased ventilator days and barotrauma.[32] The use of higher positive end-expiratory pressure in addition to low tidal volume helps minimize atelectrauma and has shown improvement in survival.[51] However, the use of low tidal volume ventilation in patients with ARDS secondary to inhalation injury can be challenging given the unique pathophysiology. Data from a pediatric study showed benefits when using higher tidal volumes.[20]

Prone positioning
Prone ventilation refers to the delivery of MV, whereas the patient is lying in the PP. This maneuver improves gas exchange by ameliorating the ventral-dorsal transpulmonary pressure difference, reducing dorsal lung compression, improving lung perfusion, and providing more homogeneous aeration of the lung.[52] The PROSEVA trial, a multicenter, prospective, randomized, controlled trial on non-burn patients with ARDS, found that in patients with P/F of less than 150 mm Hg, early prolonged PP significantly decreased 28-day and

90-day mortality.[53] Data on burn patients are limited. A case series of 18 burn patients with ARDS showed improvement in oxygenation when PP was applied.[54]

Inhaled pulmonary vasodilators

Inhaled pulmonary vasodilators selectively dilate the vessels that perfuse well-ventilated lung zones, resulting in improved oxygenation due to better ventilation/perfusion (V/Q) matching.[55] A meta-analysis of 12 trials from non-burn ARDS patients found that the usage of nitric oxide improved oxygenation without improving survival.[56] Small studies on both pediatric and adult burn patients showed improvement in oxygenation parameters.[57]

Neuromuscular blockade

Neuromuscular blockade agents (NMB) were used quite frequently in the past for patient with severe ARDS. This practice was due to the findings from the ACURASYS trial. The study showed that patients receiving NMB had a decrease in mortality, more ventilator free days and less barotrauma. Nine years later the publishing of the ROSE trial debunked that theory showing no difference in patients with severe ARDS using NMB.[58] Currently, there is no specific evidence to guide the use of NMB in burn-injured patients with ARDS, unless it is necessary for ventilator desynchrony.

Corticosteroids

The use of corticosteroids for ARDS remains controversial as there is still no consensus on its use. The ARDSnet trial, the largest trial to date, showed no difference in mortality.[59] However, when all the studies are taken together, the data suggest a probable benefit in mortality. There are no data published specific to burn patients, and for this reason, the decision to use corticosteroids must be approached carefully, weighing the risk and benefits specific to the population.

Pneumonia

The most common complication in patients with inhalation injury is pneumonia. The combination of airway injury, debris, impaired clearance of mucous, and obstruction of small airways leads to the development of pneumonia. Those with inhalation injuries are at significantly higher risk of developing pneumonia than burned without an inhalation injury. In some studies, the incidence of pneumonia in those with inhalation injury ranges from 27% to 70% with a mortality rate as high as 60%.[9,60] In a study by Liodaki and colleagues, the development of pneumonia increased length of stay (36.0 days vs 17.1 days, $P < .01$) and those with larger burns were at higher risk of developing

a pneumonia (the mean TBSA in the pneumonia group was 24.8 vs 16.9 in the non-pneumonia group, $P < .01$).[61] The investigators also found that 73.9% of patients who developed pneumonia required a tracheostomy with an average number of days on the ventilator of 25.2 days.[61]

The diagnosis of pneumonia is a combination of clinical examination, radiographic findings, and microbiologic evidence. Typically, those with pneumonia will have an elevated white blood cell count, fever, tachycardia, and purulent respiratory secretions and may have evidence of worsening respiratory status (eg, increased respiratory rate and increased ventilator requirements). It may be difficult to elucidate whether these clinical signs/symptoms and laboratory findings are indicative of infection or are normal in the setting of burn injuries, given that it is a pro-inflammatory state. A chest radiograph may assist in the diagnosis of pneumonia. The classic finding is a consolidation or infiltrate. If there is a suspicion of pneumonia, bronchoscopy and bronchoalveolar lavage can be performed to obtain cultures.

Once there is a clinical concern of pneumonia, empirical antibiotics should be started. The local antibiogram of the hospital can help guide antibiotic choice.[62–64] The most common organisms in ventilator-associated pneumonias are *Pseudomonas*, *Staphylococcus aureus*, and *Enterobacteriaceae*.[60] Cultures should be obtained to appropriately narrow antibiotics and direct therapy. Shorter courses are preferred over longer courses, typically 7 to 10 days.[65]

Exogenous Surfactant

After severe smoke inhalation injury, the lung loses its ability to protect itself through many mechanisms.[66–69] Exogenously replacing the lost surfactant has been proposed as a strategy to mitigate post-inhalation injury complications.[66,70,71] Sen and colleagues conducted a retrospective, case series ($n = 7$) of pediatric patients given inhaled calfactant 80 mL/m^2 every 12 hours for two doses and found improved oxygenation in the four patients treated early after injury.[72]

Inhaled Heparin

Originally studied in an ovine model, the use of inhaled heparin has been shown to reduce tracheobronchial cast formation, improve oxygenation, minimize barotrauma, and reduce pulmonary edema after inhalation injury.[73–75] Early small clinical studies have demonstrated mixed results, and the planned large multicenter, randomized controlled trial was halted due to difficult enrollment and high costs associated with conducted trial.[76–79] In a retrospective cohort study, inhaled unfractionated heparin (UFH) 5000 units administered during the first 72 hours failed to demonstrate a reduction in pneumonia, ventilator days, mortality, or length of stay.[80] Elsharnouby and colleagues conducted a prospective, double-blind randomized study and found inhaled UFH 10,000 units (vs 5000 units) improved lung injury scores and reduced duration of MV.[81]

Following the positive findings of their initial single-center, retrospective cohort study, Walroth and colleagues conducted a similar two-center study comparing two different dosing arms to a control group (n = 105).[82,83] The interventional treatment protocol consisted of inhaled UFH (5000 units or 10,000 units) given every 4 hours and an inhaled mucolytic (acetylcysteine or sodium bicarbonate) plus albuterol every 4 hours. Inhaled therapies were initiated on admission, alternated, and administered such that a nebulized treatment was given every 2 hours for 7 days (or until extubation, if sooner). Ventilator-free days in the first 28 days were significantly improved in the two UFH groups versus control (heparin 5000 units 22.0 ± 9.0, heparin 10,000 units 17.9 ± 7.0, control 13.6 ± 9.0; P < .001).[83] Similarly, there were significantly lower rates of ventilator-associated pneumonia and shorter lengths of stay in the groups administered inhaled UFH. Although the treatment groups were well-matched to controls based on injury severity and age and the investigators describe similar practices between centers, the analysis is limited by the retrospective design, including only two centers without controlling for potential center effect and assumptions in other aspects of clinical management. Although blood-stained sputum is common after severe smoke inhalation injury and large doses (150,000 units) of inhaled UFH have been noted to have systemic absorption over time resulting in increased activated partial thromboplastin time, doses of 10,000 units of inhaled UFH seem safe and well tolerated, as demonstrated in this large cohort and several preceding studies.[78,79,81,83]

TOXIC EXPOSURES

In cases of CO poisoning, there is reduced oxygen carrying capacity of the hemoglobin and the oxygen dissociation curve shifts to the left, leading to tissue hypoxia and subsequent organ dysfunction.[9] These patients should be placed on 100% humidified FiO_2 via non-rebreather, if not already intubated, reducing the half-life of CO from 4 hours to about 45 minutes. COHb values should be repeated hourly until the value is less than 10%,

where FiO_2 can be weaned. Depending on the degree of exposure, neurologic sequelae may persist.

CN toxicity can lead to tissue hypoxia by binding to and causing a conformational change in cytochrome-c oxidase, thereby, blocking mitochondrial respiration and the formation of adenosine triphosphate.[84] Although amyl and sodium nitrite can function as an antidote, they should be considered contraindicated in severe respiratory insufficiency, because they work as an antidote by forming methemoglobin.[84] Methemoglobin can potentiate poor oxygen delivery, as it also has a high affinity for oxygen. Sodium thiosulfate has been used successfully but is noted to have a slow onset and poor penetration into the central nervous system and mitochondria, where symptoms are most present and mechanism relies.[85–88] Hydroxocobalamin has been proposed as an effective antidote due to its rapid onset and distribution with a mechanism of directly binding CN to form cyanocobalamin to ultimately eliminate in the urine.[85,89,90] In addition, hydroxocobalamin is a nitric oxide scavenger and inhibits nitric oxide synthase, so it can produce profound hypertension over the subsequent hours.[91] Although used off-label in vasoplegia, the hypertensive effects may be less prominent in patients with shock.[92] Outside of hypertension, adverse effects can include headache, chromaturia or hyperpigmentation, and colorimetric-based laboratory inaccuracies.[91] Although some have found it efficacious, cost-effective, and well tolerated (even prehospital use), others have associated its use with higher rates of acute kidney injury.[93–102]

Mass casualty events, whether intentional or from neglect, can result in significant degrees of inhalation injuries with unknown chemical exposure.[103–107] Although toxic exposures should be a part of the differential, patients often present with overlapping symptoms.[108–110] Cases of passive exposure to chlorine gas or inappropriate handling of concentrated acids and bases are highly reported.[108,111,112]

FUTURE DIRECTIONS

There are still more pathophysiological stones to roll over. Work from the Glue Grant and more recently the SYSCOT study group has demonstrated the presence of a "genomic storm," leukocyte changes, and early transcriptomic evidence of immune pathway shutdown in severe burn injuries.[113–116] As discussed, ventilatory management of patients with varying degrees of inhalation injury and acute lung injury is still widely variable between centers and experts. There is limited evidential support for pharmacotherapeutic options beyond inhaled UFH, which may be aided by advancing technologies and epigenomic findings. Related, patients with severe inhalation injury have significantly higher odds of developing pneumonia. What roles do microbial diversity, antimicrobial exposure, or its manipulation play in outcomes or potential treatment? Bacteriophage therapy seems like a promising route for future investigation in pneumonia.[117–120] What roles should blood purification or extracorporeal organ support have in severe inhalation injury?[121–128] Can early mobilization reduce complications following inhalation injury?[129] In 2018, the American Burn Association's Cutaneous Thermal Injury and Inhalation Injury working group identified three priorities for future research: (1) airway repair mechanisms, (2) airway microbiome, and (3) biomarker identification.[130]

SUMMARY

Management of a thermal burns associated with an inhalation injury has increased the risk of mortality and morbidity in burn patients. A multidisciplinary approach consisting of physicians, nurses, therapists, pharmacists, and other key members of a burn team is necessary in optimizing outcomes. Care should be directed toward early diagnosis and referral, supportive care, airway protection with aggressive airway management, fluid resuscitation, treatment of CO, and CN poisoning and prevention/management of pneumonia. Improvements in mortality from inhalation injury are mainly due to widespread improvements in critical care rather than focused interventions for smoke inhalation.

CLINICS CARE POINTS

- Treatment of severe inhalation injuries can be complicated and should be protocolized.

- When there is suspicion of smoke inhalation with elevated carboxyhemoglobin, provide 100% oxygen to reduce the half-life of carbon monoxide.

- Diagnostic and therapeutic bronchoscopy should be routinely deployed in the initial treatment of inhalation injury.

- Severe inhalation injuries should be treated with inhaled heparin and a mucolytic plus a bronchodilator.

ACKNOWLEDGMENTS

Katherine Nearing, MD, for her excellent editorial skills.

DISCLOSURES

S.R. Velamuri is a consultant for Kerecis. Y. Ali, J. Lanfranco, P. Gupta, and D.M. Hill have received research funding and are a consultant for Medline Industries, LP and Trevena, Inc and a consultant for Access Pro Medical.

REFERENCES

1. Dries DJ, Endorf FW. Inhalation injury: epidemiology, pathology, treatment strategies. Scand J Trauma Resuscitation Emerg Med 2013;21:31.
2. Palmieri TL. Inhalation injury: research progress and needs. J Burn Care Res 2007;28(4):549–54.
3. Finland M, Davidson CS, Levenson SM. Effects of plasma and fluid on pulmonary complications in burned patients; study of the effects in the victims of the Cocoanut Grove fire. Arch Intern Med 1946; 77:477–90.
4. Pittman HS, Schatzki R. Pulmonary effects of the Cocoanut Grove fire; a 5 year follow up study. N Engl J Med 1949;241(25):1008.
5. Cancio LC. Airway management and smoke inhalation injury in the burn patient. Clin Plast Surg 2009; 36(4):555–67.
6. El-Helbawy RH, Ghareeb FM. Inhalation injury as a prognostic factor for mortality in burn patients. Ann Burns Fire Disasters 2011;24(2):82–8.
7. Bittner E, Sheridan R. Acute respiratory distress syndrome, mechanical ventilation, and inhalation injury in burn patients. Surg Clin North Am 2023; 103(3):439–51.
8. Jones SW, Williams FN, Cairns BA, et al. Inhalation injury: pathophysiology, diagnosis, and treatment. Clin Plast Surg 2017;44(3):505–11.
9. Walker PF, Buehner MF, Wood LA, et al. Diagnosis and management of inhalation injury: an updated review. Crit Care 2015;19:351.
10. Snell JA, Loh NH, Mahambrey T, et al. Clinical review: the critical care management of the burn patient. Crit Care 2013;17(5):241.
11. Marek K, Piotr W, Stanislaw S, et al. Fibreoptic bronchoscopy in routine clinical practice in confirming the diagnosis and treatment of inhalation burns. Burns 2007;33(5):554–60.
12. Hassan Z, Wong JK, Bush J, et al. Assessing the severity of inhalation injuries in adults. Burns 2010;36(2):212–6.
13. Oh JS, Chung KK, Allen A, et al. Admission chest CT complements fiberoptic bronchoscopy in prediction of adverse outcomes in thermally injured patients. J Burn Care Res 2012;33(4):532–8.
14. Yamamura H, Kaga S, Kaneda K, et al. Chest computed tomography performed on admission helps predict the severity of smoke-inhalation injury. Crit Care 2013;17(3):R95.

15. D'Avignon LC, Hogan BK, Murray CK, et al. Contribution of bacterial and viral infections to attributable mortality in patients with severe burns: an autopsy series. Burns 2010;36(6):773–9.

16. Irrazabal CL, Capdevila AA, Revich L, et al. Early and late complications among 15 victims exposed to indoor fire and smoke inhalation. Burns 2008; 34(4):533–8.

17. Shirani KZ, Pruitt BA Jr, Mason AD Jr. The influence of inhalation injury and pneumonia on burn mortality. Ann Surg 1987;205(1):82–7.

18. Endorf FW, Gamelli RL. Inhalation injury, pulmonary perturbations, and fluid resuscitation. J Burn Care Res 2007;28(1):80–3.

19. Carr JA, Phillips BD, Bowling WM. The utility of bronchoscopy after inhalation injury complicated by pneumonia in burn patients: results from the National Burn Repository. J Burn Care Res 2009; 30(6):967–74.

20. Sousse LE, Herndon DN, Andersen CR, et al. High tidal volume decreases adult respiratory distress syndrome, atelectasis, and ventilator days compared with low tidal volume in pediatric burned patients with inhalation injury. J Am Coll Surg 2015; 220(4):570–8.

21. Esnault P, Prunet B, Cotte J, et al. Tracheal intubation difficulties in the setting of face and neck burns: myth or reality? Am J Emerg Med 2014; 32(10):1174–8.

22. Dyson K, Baker P, Garcia N, et al. To intubate or not to intubate? Predictors of inhalation injury in burn-injured patients before arrival at the burn centre. Emerg Med Australas 2021;33(2):262–9.

23. Koshkareva YA, Hughes WB, Soliman AMS. Laryngotracheal stenosis in burn patients requiring mechanical ventilation. World J Otorhinolaryngol Head Neck Surg 2018;4(2):117–21.

24. Aggarwal S, Smailes S, Dziewulski P. Tracheostomy in burns patients revisited. Burns 2009; 35(7):962–6.

25. Tsuchiya A, Yamana H, Kawahara T, et al. Tracheostomy and mortality in patients with severe burns: a nationwide observational study. Burns 2018; 44(8):1954–61.

26. Saffle JR, Morris SE, Edelman L. Early tracheostomy does not improve outcome in burn patients. J Burn Care Rehabil 2002;23(6):431–8.

27. Smailes S, Spoors C, da Costa FM, et al. Early tracheostomy and active exercise programmes in adult intensive care patients with severe burns. Burns 2022;48(7):1599–605.

28. Clayton NA, Ward EC, Rumbach AF, et al. Influence of inhalation injury on incidence, clinical profile and recovery pattern of dysphagia following burn injury. Dysphagia 2020;35(6):968–77.

29. Smailes ST, Ives M, Richardson P, et al. Percutaneous dilational and surgical tracheostomy in burn patients: incidence of complications and dysphagia. Burns 2014;40(3):436–42.

30. Janik S, Grasl S, Yildiz E, et al. A new nomogram to predict the need for tracheostomy in burned patients. Eur Arch Oto-Rhino-Laryngol 2021;278(9):3479–88.

31. Amato MB, Barbas CS, Medeiros DM, et al. Effect of a protective-ventilation strategy on mortality in the acute respiratory distress syndrome. N Engl J Med 1998;338(6):347–54.

32. Acute Respiratory Distress Syndrome N, Brower RG, Matthay MA, et al. Ventilation with lower tidal volumes as compared with traditional tidal volumes for acute lung injury and the acute respiratory distress syndrome. N Engl J Med 2000;342(18):1301–8.

33. Chung KK, Rhie RY, Lundy JB, et al. A survey of mechanical ventilator practices across burn centers in North America. J Burn Care Res 2016; 37(2):e131–9.

34. Zhou Y, Jin X, Lv Y, et al. Early application of airway pressure release ventilation may reduce the duration of mechanical ventilation in acute respiratory distress syndrome. Intensive Care Med 2017; 43(11):1648–59.

35. Batchinsky AI, Burkett SE, Zanders TB, et al. Comparison of airway pressure release ventilation to conventional mechanical ventilation in the early management of smoke inhalation injury in swine. Crit Care Med 2011;39(10):2314–21.

36. Cioffi WG, Graves TA, McManus WF, et al. High-frequency percussive ventilation in patients with inhalation injury. J Trauma 1989;29(3):350–4.

37. Cioffi WG Jr, Rue LW 3rd, Graves TA, et al. Prophylactic use of high-frequency percussive ventilation in patients with inhalation injury. Ann Surg 1991; 213(6):575–80 [discussion: 580-572].

38. Chung KK, Wolf SE, Renz EM, et al. High-frequency percussive ventilation and low tidal volume ventilation in burns: a randomized controlled trial. Crit Care Med 2010;38(10):1970–7.

39. Fessler HE, Derdak S, Ferguson ND, et al. A protocol for high-frequency oscillatory ventilation in adults: results from a roundtable discussion. Crit Care Med 2007;35(7):1649–54.

40. Cartotto R, Walia G, Ellis S, et al. Oscillation after inhalation: high frequency oscillatory ventilation in burn patients with the acute respiratory distress syndrome and co-existing smoke inhalation injury. J Burn Care Res 2009;30(1):119–27.

41. Ferguson ND, Cook DJ, Guyatt GH, et al. High-frequency oscillation in early acute respiratory distress syndrome. N Engl J Med 2013;368(9):795–805.

42. Young D, Lamb SE, Shah S, et al. High-frequency oscillation for acute respiratory distress syndrome. N Engl J Med 2013;368(9):806–13.

43. Asmussen S, Maybauer DM, Fraser JF, et al. Extracorporeal membrane oxygenation in burn and smoke inhalation injury. Burns 2013;39(3):429–35.

44. Nosanov LB, McLawhorn MM, Vigiola Cruz M, et al. A national perspective on ECMO utilization use in patients with burn injury. J Burn Care Res 2017; 39(1):10–4.

45. Ware LB, Matthay MA. Clinical practice. Acute pulmonary edema. N Engl J Med 2005;353(26): 2788–96.

46. Pruitt BA Jr. Protection from excessive resuscitation: "pushing the pendulum back". J Trauma 2000;49(3):567–8.

47. Ashbaugh DG, Bigelow DB, Petty TL, et al. Acute respiratory distress in adults. Lancet 1967; 2(7511):319–23.

48. Force ADT, Ranieri VM, Rubenfeld GD, et al. Acute respiratory distress syndrome: the Berlin Definition. JAMA 2012;307(23):2526–33.

49. Belenkiy SM, Buel AR, Cannon JW, et al. Acute respiratory distress syndrome in wartime military burns: application of the Berlin criteria. J Trauma Acute Care Surg 2014;76(3):821–7.

50. Lam NN, Hung TD. ARDS among cutaneous burn patients combined with inhalation injury: early onset and bad outcome. Ann Burns Fire Disasters 2019;32(1):37–42.

51. Briel M, Meade M, Mercat A, et al. Higher vs lower positive end-expiratory pressure in patients with acute lung injury and acute respiratory distress syndrome: systematic review and meta-analysis. JAMA 2010;303(9):865–73.

52. Pelosi P, Tubiolo D, Mascheroni D, et al. Effects of the prone position on respiratory mechanics and gas exchange during acute lung injury. Am J Respir Crit Care Med 1998;157(2):387–93.

53. Guerin C, Reignier J, Richard JC, et al. Prone positioning in severe acute respiratory distress syndrome. N Engl J Med 2013;368(23):2159–68.

54. Hale DF, Cannon JW, Batchinsky AI, et al. Prone positioning improves oxygenation in adult burn patients with severe acute respiratory distress syndrome. J Trauma Acute Care Surg 2012;72(6):1634–9.

55. Rossaint R, Falke KJ, Lopez F, et al. Inhaled nitric oxide for the adult respiratory distress syndrome. N Engl J Med 1993;328(6):399–405.

56. Adhikari NK, Burns KE, Friedrich JO, et al. Effect of nitric oxide on oxygenation and mortality in acute lung injury: systematic review and meta-analysis. BMJ 2007;334(7597):779.

57. Sheridan RL, Hurford WE, Kacmarek RM, et al. Inhaled nitric oxide in burn patients with respiratory failure. J Trauma 1997;42(4):629–34.

58. National Heart L, Blood Institute PCTN, Moss M, et al. Early neuromuscular blockade in the acute respiratory distress syndrome. N Engl J Med 2019;380(21):1997–2008.

59. Steinberg KP, Hudson LD, Goodman RB, et al. Efficacy and safety of corticosteroids for persistent acute respiratory distress syndrome. N Engl J Med 2006;354(16):1671–84.

60. Brusselaers N, Logie D, Vogelaers D, et al. Inhalation injury and ventilator-associated pneumonia: value of routine surveillance cultures. Burns 2012; 38(3):364–70.

61. Liodaki E, Kalousis K, Mauss KL, et al. Epidemiology of pneumonia in a burn care unit: the influence of inhalation trauma on pneumonia and of pneumonia on burn mortality. Ann Burns Fire Disasters 2015;28(2):128–33.

62. Hill DM, Sinclair SE, Hickerson WL. Rational selection and use of antimicrobials in patients with burn injuries. Clin Plast Surg 2017;44(3):521–34.

63. Hill DM, Todor LA. Deficiencies of rule-based technology-generated antibiograms for specialized care units. Antibiotics (Basel) 2023;12(6).

64. Kalanuria AA, Ziai W, Mirski M, et al. Ventilator-associated pneumonia in the ICU. Crit Care 2014; 18(2):208.

65. Greenhalgh DGHD, Burmeister DM, Burmeister DM, et al. Surviving sepsis after burn campaign. Burns 2023;49(2).

66. Clark WR Jr, Nieman GF, Goyette D, et al. Effects of crystalloid on lung fluid balance after smoke inhalation. Ann Surg 1988;208(1):56–64.

67. Tranbaugh RF, Elings VB, Christensen JM, et al. Effect of inhalation injury on lung water accumulation. J Trauma 1983;23(7):597–604.

68. Youn YK, Lalonde C, Demling R. Oxidants and the pathophysiology of burn and smoke inhalation injury. Free Radic Biol Med 1992;12(5):409–15.

69. Clark CJ, Pollock AJ, Reid WH, et al. Role of pulmonary alveolar macrophage activation in acute lung injury after burns and smoke inhalation. Lancet 1988;2(8616):872–4.

70. Nieman GF, Clark WR Jr, Wax SD, et al. The effect of smoke inhalation on pulmonary surfactant. Ann Surg 1980;191(2):171–81.

71. Nieman GF, Paskanik AM, Fluck RR, et al. Comparison of exogenous surfactants in the treatment of wood smoke inhalation. Am J Respir Crit Care Med 1995;152(2):597–602.

72. Sen S, Tung K, Palmieri T, et al. Surfactant therapy for acute respiratory distress in severe pediatric burn injury: a case series. J Burn Care Res 2012; 33(2):e88–91.

73. Cox CS Jr, Zwischenberger JB, Traber DL, et al. Heparin improves oxygenation and minimizes barotrauma after severe smoke inhalation in an ovine model. Surg Gynecol Obstet 1993;176(4):339–49.

74. Murakami K, McGuire R, Cox RA, et al. Heparin nebulization attenuates acute lung injury in sepsis following smoke inhalation in sheep. Shock 2002; 18(3):236–41.

75. Tasaki O, Mozingo DW, Dubick MA, et al. Effects of heparin and lisofylline on pulmonary function after

smoke inhalation injury in an ovine model. Crit Care Med 2002;30(3):637–43.

76. Glas GJ, Serpa Neto A, Horn J, et al. Nebulized heparin for patients under mechanical ventilation: an individual patient data meta-analysis. Ann Intensive Care 2016;6(1):33.

77. Glas GJ, Muller J, Binnekade JM, et al. Hepburn - investigating the efficacy and safety of nebulized heparin versus placebo in burn patients with inhalation trauma: study protocol for a multi-center randomized controlled trial. Trials 2014;15:91.

78. Glas GJ, Horn J, Binnekade JM, et al. Nebulized heparin in burn patients with inhalation trauma-safety and feasibility. J Clin Med 2020;9(4).

79. Miller AC, Elamin EM, Suffredini AF. Inhaled anticoagulation regimens for the treatment of smoke inhalation-associated acute lung injury: a systematic review. Crit Care Med 2014;42(2):413–9.

80. Holt J, Saffle JR, Morris SE, et al. Use of inhaled heparin/N-acetylcystine in inhalation injury: does it help? J Burn Care Res 2008;29(1):192–5.

81. Elsharnouby NM, Eid HE, Abou Elezz NF, et al. Heparin/N-acetylcysteine: an adjuvant in the management of burn inhalation injury: a study of different doses. J Crit Care 2014;29(1):182 e181–e184.

82. McIntire AM, Harris SA, Whitten JA, et al. Outcomes following the use of nebulized heparin for inhalation injury (HIHI study). J Burn Care Res 2017;38(1):45–52.

83. Cox CL, McIntire AM, Bolton KJ, et al. A multicenter evaluation of outcomes following the use of nebulized heparin for inhalation injury (HIHI2 study). J Burn Care Res 2020;41(5):1004–8.

84. Lawson-Smith P, Jansen EC, Hyldegaard O. Cyanide intoxication as part of smoke inhalation–a review on diagnosis and treatment from the emergency perspective. Scand J Trauma Resuscitation Emerg Med 2011;19:14.

85. Way JL. Cyanide intoxication and its mechanism of antagonism. Annu Rev Pharmacol Toxicol 1984;24:451–81.

86. Piantadosi CA, Sylvia AL. Cerebral cytochrome a,a3 inhibition by cyanide in bloodless rats. Toxicology 1984;33(1):67–79.

87. Morocco AP. Cyanides. Crit Care Clin 2005;21(4):691–705, vi.

88. Baskin SI, Horowitz AM, Nealley EW. The antidotal action of sodium nitrite and sodium thiosulfate against cyanide poisoning. J Clin Pharmacol 1992;32(4):368–75.

89. Hall AH, Saiers J, Baud F. Which cyanide antidote? Crit Rev Toxicol 2009;39(7):541–52.

90. Forsyth JC, Mueller PD, Becker CE, et al. Hydroxocobalamin as a cyanide antidote: safety, efficacy and pharmacokinetics in heavily smoking normal volunteers. J Toxicol Clin Toxicol 1993;31(2):277–94.

91. Shapeton AD, Mahmood F, Ortoleva JP. Hydroxocobalamin for the treatment of vasoplegia: a review of current literature and considerations for use. J Cardiothorac Vasc Anesth 2019;33(4):894–901.

92. Ritter LA, Maldarelli M, McCurdy MT, et al. Effects of a single bolus of hydroxocobalamin on hemodynamics in vasodilatory shock. J Crit Care 2022;67:66–71.

93. Borron SW, Baud FJ, Barriot P, et al. Prospective study of hydroxocobalamin for acute cyanide poisoning in smoke inhalation. Ann Emerg Med 2007;49(6):794–801, 801 e791-e792.

94. Dumestre D, Nickerson D. Use of cyanide antidotes in burn patients with suspected inhalation injuries in North America: a cross-sectional survey. J Burn Care Res 2014;35(2):e112–7.

95. Purvis MV, Rooks H, Young Lee J, et al. Prehospital hydroxocobalamin for inhalation injury and cyanide toxicity in the United States - analysis of a database and survey of EMS providers. Ann Burns Fire Disasters 2017;30(2):126–8.

96. Nguyen L, Afshari A, Kahn SA, et al. Utility and outcomes of hydroxocobalamin use in smoke inhalation patients. Burns 2017;43(1):107–13.

97. Engwall AJ, Blache A, Lintner A, et al. Hydroxocobalamin administration after inhalation injury is not associated with mesenteric ischemia. Ann Burns Fire Disasters 2021;34(3):240–4.

98. Sanders KN, Aggarwal J, Stephens JM, et al. Cost impact of hydroxocobalamin in the treatment of patients with known or suspected cyanide poisoning due to smoke inhalation from closed-space fires. Burns 2022;48(6):1325–30.

99. Hamdini L, Ydee A, Larsen S, et al. Hydroxocobalamin-induced oxalate nephropathy after smoke inhalation. J Nephrol 2023.

100. Pruskowski KA, Britton GW, Cancio LC. Outcomes after the administration of hydroxocobalamin. Int J Burns Trauma 2020;10(5):231–6.

101. Depret F, Hoffmann C, Daoud L, et al. Association between hydroxocobalamin administration and acute kidney injury after smoke inhalation: a multicenter retrospective study. Crit Care 2019;23(1):421.

102. Legrand M, Michel T, Daudon M, et al. Risk of oxalate nephropathy with the use of cyanide antidote hydroxocobalamin in critically ill burn patients. Intensive Care Med 2016;42(6):1080–1.

103. Madsen JM. Toxins as weapons of mass destruction. A comparison and contrast with biological-warfare and chemical-warfare agents. Clin Lab Med 2001;21(3):593–605.

104. Baker DJ. The pre-hospital management of injury following mass toxic release; a comparison of military and civil approaches. Resuscitation 1999;42(2):155–9.

105. Turris SA, Lund A, Bowles RR. An analysis of mass casualty incidents in the setting of mass gatherings

and special events. Disaster Med Public Health Prep 2014;8(2):143–9.

106. Leclerc T, Sjoberg F, Jennes S, et al. European Burns Association guidelines for the management of burn mass casualty incidents within a European response plan. Burns 2023;49(2):275–303.

107. Cheng MH, Mathews AL, Chuang SS, et al. Management of the formosa color dust explosion: lessons learned from the treatment of 49 mass burn casualty patients at Chang Gung Memorial Hospital. Plast Reconstr Surg 2016;137(6):1900–8.

108. Pascuzzi TA, Storrow AB. Mass casualties from acute inhalation of chloramine gas. Mil Med 1998; 163(2):102–4.

109. Peck B, Workeneh B, Kadikoy H, et al. Spectrum of sodium hypochlorite toxicity in man-also a concern for nephrologists. NDT Plus 2011;4(4):231–5.

110. Pavelites JJ, Kemp WL, Barnard JJ, et al. Deaths related to chemical burns. Am J Forensic Med Pathol 2011;32(4):387–92.

111. Sexton JD, Pronchik DJ. Chlorine inhalation: the big picture. J Toxicol Clin Toxicol 1998;36(1–2):87–93.

112. Wilken JA, DiMaggio M, Kaufmann M, et al. Inhalational chlorine injuries at public aquatic venues - California, 2008-2015. MMWR Morb Mortal Wkly Rep 2017;66(19):498–501.

113. Sood RF, Gibran NS, Arnoldo BD, et al. Early leukocyte gene expression associated with age, burn size, and inhalation injury in severely burned adults. J Trauma Acute Care Surg 2016;80(2): 250–7.

114. Xiao W, Mindrinos MN, Seok J, et al. A genomic storm in critically injured humans. J Exp Med 2011;208(13):2581–90.

115. Tompkins RG. Genomics of injury: the Glue grant experience. J Trauma Acute Care Surg 2015; 78(4):671–86.

116. Keyloun JW, Campbell R, Carney BC, et al. Early transcriptomic response to burn injury: severe burns are associated with immune pathway shutdown. J Burn Care Res 2022;43(2):306–14.

117. Tamma PD, Souli M, Billard M, et al. Safety and microbiological activity of phage therapy in persons with cystic fibrosis colonized with Pseudomonas aeruginosa: study protocol for a phase 1b/2, multicenter, randomized, double-blind, placebo-controlled trial. Trials 2022;23(1):1057.

118. Plumet L, Ahmad-Mansour N, Dunyach-Remy C, et al. Bacteriophage therapy for Staphylococcus aureus infections: a review of animal models,

treatments, and clinical trials. Front Cell Infect Microbiol 2022;12:907314.

119. Herridge WP, Shibu P, O'Shea J, et al. Bacteriophages of Klebsiella spp., their diversity and potential therapeutic uses. J Med Microbiol 2020; 69(2):176–94.

120. Tagliaferri TL, Jansen M, Horz HP. Fighting pathogenic bacteria on two fronts: phages and antibiotics as combined strategy. Front Cell Infect Microbiol 2019;9:22.

121. Ronco C, Bagshaw SM, Bellomo R, et al. Extracorporeal blood purification and organ support in the critically ill patient during COVID-19 pandemic: expert review and recommendation. Blood Purif 2021;50(1):17–27.

122. Monard C, Abraham P, Schneider A, et al. New targets for extracorporeal blood purification therapies in sepsis. Blood Purif 2023;52(1):1–7.

123. Chung KK, Coates EC, Smith DJ Jr, et al. High-volume hemofiltration in adult burn patients with septic shock and acute kidney injury: a multicenter randomized controlled trial. Crit Care 2017;21(1): 289.

124. Chung KK, Coates EC, Hickerson WL, et al. Renal replacement therapy in severe burns: a multicenter observational study. J Burn Care Res 2018;39(6): 1017–21.

125. Hill DM, Rizzo JA, Aden JK, et al. Continuous venovenous hemofiltration is associated with improved survival in burn patients with shock: a subset analysis of a multicenter observational study. Blood Purif 2021;50(4–5):473–80.

126. Yan J, Zhang Y, Zhang J. Clinical efficacy of blood purification in the treatment of sepsis: a meta-analysis of the last 5 years. Clin Lab 2023;69(6).

127. Zaky S, El Badry M, Makhlouf HA, et al. Hemofiltration as an alternative for IL-6 inhibitors in COVID-19 cytokines storm associated with underlaying bacterial infections: a review Article. Infect Disord: Drug Targets 2023.

128. Morin L, Charbel R, Cousin VL, et al. Blood purification with oXiris(c) in critically ill children with vasoplegic shock. Blood Purif 2023;1–8.

129. Cartotto R, Johnson L, Rood JM, et al. Clinical practice guideline: early mobilization and rehabilitation of critically ill burn patients. J Burn Care Res 2023;44(1):1–15.

130. Dyamenahalli K, Garg G, Shupp JW, et al. Inhalation injury: unmet clinical needs and future research. J Burn Care Res 2019;40(5):570–84.

Surgical Excision of Burn Wounds

Anjali C. Raghuram, MD[a], Guy M. Stofman, MD[a], Jenny A. Ziembicki, MD[b], Francesco M. Egro, MD, MSc, MRCS[a,b],*

KEYWORDS

• Burn wound • Surgical debridement • Burn excision

KEY POINTS

- Burn wound excision is performed to improve patient survival, functional recovery, and aesthetic results.
- Excision is performed tangentially or down to fascia, with use of hemostatic techniques and agents to minimize intraoperative blood loss.
- Specialized anatomic regions, including the face, breast, hands, and perianal and genital regions, require consideration of aesthetic subunits, judicious excision to minimize and treat scarring, and infection prevention.
- Postoperative patient care relies on topical dressings and treatments, wound cleansing, pain control, and nutritional supplementation.

INTRODUCTION

Over the last few decades, advances in the understanding of burn injury and surgical treatment have enabled a multifaceted approach in the care of these patients. With collaboration among plastic and general surgery, critical care, anesthesiology, nursing staff, the nutrition team, occupational and physical therapy, social work, pharmacy, and other individuals invested in burn care, there has been remarkable improvement in the treatment of burn patients from presentation at hospitals and burn centers to their outpatient follow-up visits.[1] Burn injuries affect patients of all ages and can involve skin and/or deeper structures. Of critical importance is the timing of surgical excision and coverage of these burn wounds to ensure optimal outcomes with respect to patient survival, function, and aesthetics.[2]

The practice of thoughtful and timely surgical debridement and burn wound coverage has improved patient morbidity and mortality.[3]

Following the initial stabilization of a patient presenting with burn injury, urgent surgical procedures for life and limb preservation, including escharotomies and fasciotomies, precede burn wound excision. The often iterative process of burn wound excision focuses on the debridement of burnt tissue, while attempting to maintain dermal vascularity and integrity when possible, to improve wound healing and minimize scar burden.[2,3] When deciding the optimal time to perform burn surgical procedures, a balance is sought in terms of avoiding hypermetabolism and catabolism while ensuring the patient is stable to undergo serial debridements with blood loss and temperature derangement.[3] However, the gold standard is early burn excision and wound coverage, which can result in improvements in patient mortality, hospital stay length, and functional and cosmetic outcomes.[4] A survey of the American Burn Association demonstrated that 56% of surgeons perform excision as early as Day 1 postinjury and 73% of surgeons excise greater than

[a] Department of Plastic Surgery, University of Pittsburgh Medical Center, Pittsburgh, PA, USA; [b] Department of Surgery, University of Pittsburgh Medical Center, Pittsburgh, PA, USA
* Corresponding author. Department of Plastic Surgery, University of Pittsburgh Medical Center, 1350 Locust Street, Medical Professional Building, Suite G103, Pittsburgh, PA 15219.
E-mail address: francescoegro@gmail.com

Clin Plastic Surg 51 (2024) 233–240
https://doi.org/10.1016/j.cps.2023.11.002

20% of total body surface area (TBSA) comprised by these burn wounds in one setting.[5] A recent study by De La Tejera and colleagues[6] reviewed 6158 burn patients that underwent wound excision within 14 days of burn injury. The authors found a significantly lower risk of mortality in patients who underwent excision within the first 3 days (3.84%) as compared with 8 to 14 days after the burn (6.09%; $P < .05$), a decreased risk of wound infection in patients who underwent excision within 0 to 3 days (37.84%) as compared with 4 to 7 days after the burn (42.48%; $P < .05$), and a significantly decreased risk of hypertrophic scarring in patients who underwent excision within 0 to 3 days (22%) as compared with 4 to 7 days (28%; $P < .05$). Although other studies have showed an increase in blood transfusion requirements with early excision, De La Tejera and colleagues showed no difference in blood transfusion requirements between early versus more delayed timing of excision.[6,7]

All patients with a burn injury should have their wounds evaluated for degree and depth of injury. An assessment of burn wound depth determines whether wounds will heal spontaneously or require surgical management. This assessment is performed clinically or with the use of technological diagnostic tools. Clinical parameters to qualify skin viability include color and capillary refill, sensation, presence or absence of epidermal appendages postinjury, and blistering.[3] Laser Doppler flowmetry and infrared thermography are diagnostic tools that may be used to complement and confirm clinical judgment of burn wound depth. Burn wounds evolve over time and if the clinical picture is uncertain, one needs to allow the burn to declare itself fully over a few days.

Superficial burns (superficial and superficial partial-thickness) do not compromise dermal integrity and therefore heal largely by self-regeneration. In contrast, deep partial-thickness or full-thickness burn injuries are characterized by lack of adequate blood supply and epidermal appendages that harbor stem cells required for wound healing. These latter types of wounds benefit from surgical excision. In addition to wound depth, the TBSA of burn injury influences duration of surgical debridement and dictates how injuries need to be sequentially addressed in order of anatomic location (ie, anterior vs posterior, dorsal vs volar).[3]

In some scenarios, assessing burn depth visually is imprecise and these wounds are categorized as indeterminate depth burns (IDBs). These injuries are challenging to manage because their healing capacity is uncertain, as is the potential to be augmented by conservative and surgical wound care measures. Similar to deep partial-thickness or second-degree burns, IDBs may involve the epidermis or deep dermis, result in gross erythema or pale skin with blistering, and be painful or anesthetic, without blanching on application of pressure.[8] Unlike second-degree burns, IDBs can involve the full dermis and have a healing time that is likely longer than 2 to 3 weeks. Although posing an initial diagnostic uncertainty, IDBs are managed akin to second- and third-degree burns, with timely debridement and wound coverage.

SURGICAL TECHNIQUES

Burn wound excision is performed in either a tangential or fascial manner. Tangential excision was first described by Janzekovic[9] in 1970 as an evolutionary technique from fascial excision. This entails sequential excision slices to remove burned, nonviable tissue down to healthy vascularized tissue (Figs. 1A–D and 2). Deep partial-thickness burns are excised down to white viable dermis with punctate bleeding. Full-thickness burns are excised down to viable tissue: yellow glistening fat, glistening fascia, or sometimes down to bone. In very deep burns, a burr might be required to debride necrotic periosteum and bone cortex. Indications that incomplete excision has been performed include presence of necrotic tissue; lack of punctate bleeding; a dull, yellow fat color; and presence of thrombosed vessels.

Fascial excision is a full-thickness removal of skin and subcutaneous tissue down to the muscular fascia (Fig. 3). This technique is reserved for larger, life-threatening burns that benefit from rapid excision or very deep, full-thickness burns with minimal residual fat.[10] Unlike the more judicious approach with tangential excision, fascial excision creates contour deformities, permanently alters cutaneous sensation, and carries a risk of lymphedema because of removal of lymphatics with this depth of excision.

An array of instruments may be used for performing burn debridement and tangential/fascial excision. A Norsen blade is used to remove pseudoeschar or eschar mechanically before more formal excision. Tangential excision may then be carried out with hand-held knives, including the Weck, Watson, Goulian, Braithwaite, or Humby blades (Fig. 4).

The patient's skin should be stretched with adequate tension to permit a smooth, back-and-forth motion with these blades to sequentially reach a layer of viable tissue. While excising, hemostasis is facilitated with use of Bovie electrocautery.[10] For wounds that are more superficial or smaller in size,

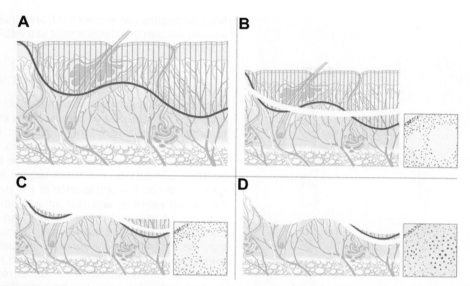

Fig. 1. (*A–D*) Schematic representation of tangential excision; sequential excision is performed down to punctate hemorrhage and healthy vascularized tissue. (*From* Janzekovic Z. A new concept in the early excision and immediate grafting of burns. J Trauma. 1970 Dec;10(12):1103–1108).

hydrodissectors, such as the Versajet (Smith & Nephew, London, UK), can debride similarly to tangential excision. Hydrosurgery provides debridement while facilitating hemostasis. Pressurized saline is injected at a high velocity into the operative field, using the Venturri effect to create a local vacuum. Placing the hand piece of the hydrodissector parallel to the wound allows for deeper excision, whereas oblique positioning permits gentler vacuuming of contaminants.[3]

Other debridement techniques include use of ultrasound technology and shock waves. A powered ultrasound device functions to promote wound healing by dispersing bacterial biofilm, decreasing wound exudate and slough, and removing chronic granulating tissue and pseudoeschar.[3] Enzymatic

debridement becomes particularly useful for patients who are unable to undergo general anesthesia caused by underlying comorbidities or coagulopathy. Although several enzymatic agents have been tested over the years for burn wound debridement, including papain, organic and inorganic acids, and bacterial proteolytic enzymes, these products' limited efficacy with increased wound depth, nonspecific action, and adverse side effects have curbed their use.[11] Collagenase has been applied since the 1940s, with favorable properties of targeting necrotic tissue without injuring nearby healthy tissue and efficacy in partial-thickness burns that are less than 25% TBSA.

A newer enzymatic agent, bromelain (Nexobrid, Mediwound, Ltd, Yavne, Israel), has demonstrated some promise in treating deeper burn wounds, reducing time needed for completion of debridement, and with resultantly improved functional and cosmetic outcomes.[11] Bromelain is derived from pineapple stem extract and has been applied for treating more than 10,000 patients thus far.[12]

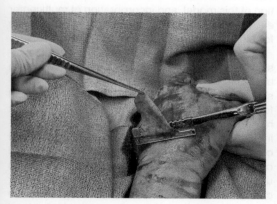

Fig. 2. Tangential excision of a mixed deep partial-thickness and full-thickness burn using a Goulian knife.

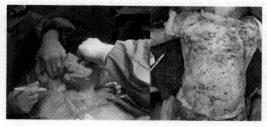

Fig. 3. Fascial excision of full-thickness burns of the trunk and bilateral upper extremities.

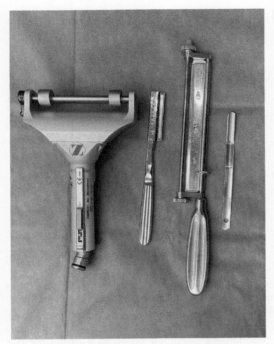

Fig. 4. Common surgical instruments used in burn surgery: dermatome, Weck knife, Humby knife, Norsen debrider (from *left* to *right*).

from the healthy yellow construct, and coagulated vessels ensures that debridement to a viable plane is achieved.

STRATEGIES TO MINIMIZE BLOOD LOSS

Burn wound excision causes considerable hemorrhage, so maintenance of hemostasis is essential to preserve the patient's hemodynamic stability and limit perioperative blood transfusions. Tourniquets and tumescent infiltration may be used to facilitate hemostasis, but these require the surgeon to rely on the appearance of the dermis or fat, vessel patency, and lack of ecchymosis as markers of tissue viability rather than simply considering punctate bleeding.[10] Tumescence may be infiltrated via a syringe manually or a pump device, with the latter resulting in reduced volume of tumescent fluid required to reach the desired end point, operative time, and improved economy of motion.[15] After excision has been performed to an acceptable level, compression and epinephrine-soaked gauze may be applied to promote hemostasis. Bovie electrocautery may be used to obtain bleeding control of larger vessels.

Intraoperative transfusion practices are correlated with extent of wound excision and the patient's complete blood count and coagulation profile on the day of surgery. Because estimates of intraoperative blood loss are subjective and vary, blood product ordering preoperatively tends to underestimate resuscitation need. Rizzo and colleagues[16] developed a predictive model for blood product ordering based on a single institution experience of 563 operations. These authors propose that small burns less than 3% TBSA require one unit of packed red blood cells, 3% to 12% TBSA burns require two units, 12% to 20% TBSA burns require three units, and 20% to 60% TBSA burns require four units. Prospective validation of this model, and incorporation of multicenter experiences, will further substantiate the evidence for blood product ordering and administration.

Skin grafting procedures after burn wound excision produce further coagulopathy, which is often unable to be corrected by blood product transfusion alone. Tranexamic acid (TXA) may be useful for decreasing blood loss in patients who do not have cardiovascular, ocular, or neurologic contraindications to use of this product. A randomized controlled trial of 30 patients by Ajai and colleagues[17] demonstrated less blood loss when using TXA (TXA = 258.7 ± 124.10 mL; control = 388.1 ± 173.9 mL; P = .07), and none of these TXA-treated patients required blood transfusions. Farny and colleagues[18] considered a smaller population size of 139 patients to

When compared with transitional burn excision, bromelain has superior preservation of normal tissue, resulting in satisfactory debridement and wound optimization for closure. Of note, there are no significant differences with respect to scar formation when comparing bromelain and traditional surgical debridement.[13] Nonetheless, patients report increased satisfaction with this enzymatic debridement because of concomitant analgesic protocols, reduced need for further operative interventions including autologous skin grafting, and reduced length of hospital stay.[14] Favorable receipt of bromelain has also resulted in its off-label application for treating facial, pediatric, and greater than 15% TBSA burns with demonstrated safety and efficacy.[14]

When performing excision, tissue viability is determined by evaluating for patent blood flow. Punctate bleeding is a helpful indicator of tissue viability, but the quality of bleeding differs based on dermal depth. Capillaries in the papillary dermis are closer together than the spaced apart arterioles in the reticular dermis.[10] In the dermal layer, excision should be performed to appreciate a white, pearly dermis and an absence of ecchymosis. When burn injury involves deeper debridement to the subcutaneous fat, meticulous removal of ecchymotic tissue, gray or brown fat that differs propose a formula for postoperative hemoglobin (Hb) estimation, such that postoperative Hb = (1- (blood loss/estimated blood volume)) * preoperative Hb. This formula assumes an estimated blood volume of 65 mL/kg for women and 70 mL/kg for men. Although attempts to improve quantification of intraoperative blood loss with burn wound excision are important, the need for transfusion should not be overestimated because overtransfusion has its own deleterious effects.

APPROACH OF SPECIALIZED ANATOMIC AREAS

Although the principles of burn wound excision tend to be uniform across the body, there are some anatomic regions that merit special consideration. The face usually has a good prognosis because it is highly vascular with great healing potential, and therefore these injuries can simply be monitored and treated conservatively. Furthermore, the face dissipates heat quickly because of its high vascularity, resulting in primarily superficial or partial-thickness burns that are treated with local wound care for spontaneous healing. Early debridement with a Norsen blade can indicate whether the skin will heal well and withstand delayed grafting. Friedstat and Klein[19] at the University of Washington perform excision of all facial burns unlikely to heal within 3 weeks of injury. Deeper facial burns and those in hair-bearing areas carry a risk of hypertrophic scarring. For facial burns that are definitely full-thickness in nature, excision is considered as soon as edema has improved.

The surgical approach to facial burn wound excision and grafting is performed in recognition of the aesthetic subunits. Deep eyelid burns can lead to severe ectropion, infection, corneal exposure, and compromised vision.[1] For this reason early excision and grafting should be considered for clear full-thickness burns. Alternatively, in the eventuality that patients develop eyelid contractures, these need to be released and grafted as soon as possible. When excising the medial canthal area, sharp iris scissors, a number 15 scalpel blade, or Versajet water dissector may facilitate careful excision.[19] The nose, upper and lower lips, and chin are approached next, following a shallow excision approach to preserve the intricacies of these structures. Lastly, the cheeks, forehead, and neck are considered. Eyebrow hairs are preserved as much as possible when excising nearby burns. Burn excision of facial burns is carried out in a tangential fashion with a knife (eg, Weck knife) to preserve most dermal elements and minimize aesthetic compromise. Excluding the eyebrow area, hair follicles should be removed in their entirety before grafting, because hair protrusion through grafts promotes infection and inflammation to cause graft loss, folliculitis, and hypertrophic scarring.[1] Ears are another challenging area in the face to manage. Cartilage exposure and infection is of concern, and thus topical antipseudomonal coverage (eg, sulfamylon cream) should be provided during the healing phase. The ears are not well-suited for tangential excision because of their shape, and aggressive debridement should be avoided unless necessary in attempt to maintain the native shape and form. If cartilage exposure develops, small areas of cartilage are excised to allow for subsequent skin grafting.[19]

Management of breast burn wounds is contingent on preservation of any viable breast bud tissue. Restricting burn scars should be excised for contracture release and followed by skin grafting. Breast envelope reconstruction is considered when the envelope is insufficient to permit unrestricted breast development. Some patients require breast mound reconstruction with musculocutaneous flaps or tissue expanders, and the contralateral breast may benefit from reduction or mastopexy, if unaffected by the initial burn injury. Nipple areolar reconstruction is undertaken after a period of compression therapy and scar settling that ranges from 6 to 12 months.[20]

The hands are of significant functional importance. The dorsal and palmar skin have different characteristics relevant to burn surgical management. The dorsal skin is thin and pliable, with a very thin subcutaneous layer separating the skin from the tendons, bone, and joints. In contrast, the palmar skin is thick and glabrous, which is strongly attached to the underlying fascia by numerous vertical fibers and contains a high concentration of sensory nerve organs. The thickness and different characteristics between the two explain why the dorsal aspect of the hand is usually more affected by burns, and the palmar aspect requires excision less frequently and portends a better prognosis. Deep burns require early excision and grafting to prevent contracture and expedite initiation of range of motion therapy.[10] Dermal substitutes, such as Integra, may be applied to excised hand burn wounds with delayed grafting to achieve reasonable functional and cosmetic outcomes.[21]

The genital and perianal regions are uncommonly burned but when severe, have devastating consequences for the patient's physical and psychological health. Genital burns often occur in conjunction with scald or extended burn injuries of the groin and perineal regions. Perianal burns are susceptible to contamination so rectal diversion with a tube is performed before debridement.[10] For pediatric patients with a better healing propensity than their adult counterparts, conservative burn treatment with loose debridement and topical or parenteral antibiotics is recommended. Surgical debridement and skin grafting is reserved for severe scrotal, testicular, or deeper genital burns. For adults with a partial-thickness or deep dermal genital or perianal burn, early surgical debridement can promote favorable aesthetic and functional results. Circumferential penile burns should be managed by removing all vital penile skin distal to the injury to prevent development of lymphedema, whereas burns of the penile glans should not be excised unless necrotic.[22] Urethral catheterization has been debated because of risk of bacterial colonization but is selectively used in cases of circumferential genital injury that requires urethral stenting.[22] Notably, urethral catheters should not be used for patients with full-thickness burns of the ventral glans and penile shaft, because these patients are better treated with a suprapubic tube that prevents pressure necrosis and severe hypospadias development.[10]

RECOMMENDATIONS FOR POSTOPERATIVE CARE

Burn wound patients should be carefully monitored for injury sequelae before and after surgical interventions. Burn injury results in hypermetabolism that exceeds that of many other surgical and traumatic conditions, necessitating regulation of thermohomeostasis, mitigation of the patient's pain and anxiety, and early burn wound closure to curtail this response and prevent infection and sepsis.[3] To prevent infection, topical treatments, such as honey, silver-impregnated dressings, and wound vacuum therapy may be applied in rotation to decrease bacterial contamination and wound metalloproteinases.[23] Topical therapies are complemented and augmented by periodic wound cleansing and antibiotic therapy that is tailored to wound cultures.

Debridement is serially performed to create burn wounds amenable to definitive coverage. During this process, temporary coverage is created with homografts or xenografts. A routine and ongoing assessment of the patient's pain should be performed, with NMDA receptor antagonists as a helpful backbone of analgesia, along with nonpharmacologic therapies. Lastly, proper nutritional support is critical throughout the perioperative burn wound management period to prevent muscle wasting, aid rehabilitation, and improve burn wound and autograft donor site healing. Early enteral feeds consist of high protein and carbohydrate formulas to decrease bacterial translocation across compromised gut-blood barriers and increase amino acid delivery to muscles. Anabolic agents, such as growth hormone, oxandrolone, and insulin, also help maintain muscle mass.[3]

FUTURE DIRECTIONS

Although the past century has observed remarkable advances in burn wound management, there are many novel developments on the horizon for improving care of these patients. Burn wound excision is performed in a timely manner but can be aggressive when guided by the surgeon's gross visual assessment alone. Overexcision of burn wounds compromises wound healing potential. Zajac and colleagues[24] addressed this challenge by studying second window indocyanine green fluorescence imaging to identify burn wound necrosis and provide an interface of viable and nonviable tissue to guide excision. These authors validated the technique in preclinical mouse skin and human xenograft models, demonstrating that second window indocyanine green fluorescent signaling and cellular necrosis overlap and can delineate the extent of surgical excision. Gupta and colleagues[25] studied the coverage of large burn wounds with limited donor skin by evaluating maximal skin graft expansion potential with novel auxetic patterns. After wound excision to a viable level, skin grafts expanded with these patterns can offer significantly greater coverage without risk of rupture when subject to uniaxial and biaxial tensile strains.[25]

Burn wound excision is timed to mitigate local and systemic immunomodulatory and inflammatory responses. However, it is important to consider how often the theory translates into clinical practice. A large retrospective, 3-year review of 1494 patients within the German burn registry revealed that less than 50% of patients underwent surgical excision within 72 hours of admission. Notably, admission on an early weekday between Sunday and Wednesday and higher TBSA correlated with earlier excision. Logistical constraints in terms of burn unit and surgical team staffing, on-call periods, and operative room availability contributed to delays in surgical intervention.[26] In a similar vein of study, a 2015 survey of members of the American Burn Association found that geographic location, board certification, individual surgeon preferences, and burn unit size contributed to variations in practice, including timing of first excision and adoption of new technologies.[26] In sum, these findings call for a more granular evaluation of how burn center and institutional practices are carried out across countries to optimize timing and extent of burn excision.

SUMMARY

Timely surgical debridement and excision of burn wounds have resulted in improvements in patient morbidity and mortality. Techniques for excision can vary based on depth achieved, tools used, and incorporation of adjunctive modalities to facilitate minimal scarring and improved hemostasis. Nevertheless, the goals of excision are consistent, in that wounds should be optimized from a tissue viability and healing standpoint to facilitate new skin growth through autografting, allografting, or native epithelialization. Coordinated multidisciplinary efforts further improve burn patient care throughout the perioperative period and merit efforts for standardizing these practices across institutions.

CLINICS CARE POINTS

- Timing of surgical excision and burn wound coverage determine patient outcomes with respect to survival, functional recovery, and aesthetics.[2]

- Timing of burn surgical procedures is achieved through a balance of avoiding patient hypermetabolic and catabolic activity and maintaining patient stability during inevitable operative blood loss and temperature derangement.[3]

- Skin viability within burn wounds is determined based on color and capillary refill, presence or absence of sensation, epidermal appendages, and blistering.[3]

- Burn wounds are excised either tangentially or down to fascia. The former removes nonviable tissue for subsequent skin grafting. The latter involves a full-thickness excision of skin and subcutaneous tissue, generally in the case of larger, life-threatening burns.[10]

- Hemostasis during burn excision is facilitated through tourniquet usage, tumescence, Bovie electrocautery, and tailored intraoperative transfusion.[10]

- Facial burn wound excision is performed by considering aesthetic subunits, with a sequence of treating the eyelids, nose, upper and lower lips, chin, and lastly the cheeks, forehead, and neck.[19]

- Breast burn scars are excised to prevent contracture, with subsequent breast envelope and mound reconstruction if the residual tissue is insufficient. Nipple areolar reconstruction is delayed until after compression therapy and scar maturation.[20]

- Deep partial- and full-thickness hand burns are excised tangentially and then may be reconstructed with dermal substitutes.[21]

- Genital and perianal burns are approached with rectal diversion, debridement and skin grafting for severe burns, and selection of urethral versus suprapubic catheterization.[10]

- Postoperative burn wound care involves antimicrobial dressings and topical treatments, wound hygiene, effective analgesia, and nutritional optimization.3,22

DISCLOSURE

The authors have no relevant commercial or financial conflicts of interest or funding sources.

REFERENCES

1. Mosier MJ, Gibran NS. Surgical excision of the burn wound. Clin Plast Surg 2009;36(4):617–25.
2. Levi B, Chan R. Principles of burn reconstruction. In: Chung KC, editor. Grabb and Smith's plastic surgery. Philadelphia, PA: Wolters Kluwer Health; 2020.
3. Leon-Villapalos J, Barret JP. Surgical repair of the acute burn wound: who, when, what techniques? What is the future? J Burn Care Res 2023; 44(Supplement_1):S5–12.
4. Miroshnychenko A, Kim K, Rochwerg B, et al. Comparison of early surgical intervention to delayed surgical intervention for treatment of thermal burns in adults: a systematic review and meta-analysis. Burns Open 2021;5(2):67–77.
5. Israel JS, Greenhalgh DG, Gibson AL. Variations in burn excision and grafting: a survey of the American Burn Association. J Burn Care Res 2017;38(1): e125–32.
6. De La Tejera G, Corona K, Efejuku T, et al. Early wound excision within three days decreases risks of wound infection and death in burned patients. Burns 2023;49(8):1816–22.
7. Ong YS, Samuel M, Song C. Meta-analysis of early excision of burns. Burns 2006;32(2):145–50.
8. Karim AS, Shaum K, Gibson ALF. Indeterminate-depth burn injury-exploring the uncertainty. J Surg Res 2020;245:183–97.
9. Janzekovic Z. A new concept in the early excision and immediate grafting of burns. J Trauma 1970; 10(12):1103–8.
10. Daugherty THF, Ross A, Neumeister MW. Surgical excision of burn wounds: best practices using evidence-based medicine. Clin Plast Surg 2017; 44(3):619–25.

11. Salehi SH, Momeni M, Vahdani M, et al. Clinical value of debriding enzymes as an adjunct to standard early surgical excision in human burns: a systematic review. J Burn Care Res 2020;41(6): 1224–30.

12. Shoham Y, Gasteratos K, Singer AJ, et al. Bromelain-based enzymatic burn debridement: A systematic review of clinical studies on patient safety, efficacy and long-term outcomes. Int Wound J 2023;20(10): 4364–83.

13. Schulz A, Shoham Y, Rosenberg L, et al. Enzymatic versus traditional surgical debridement of severely burned hands: a comparison of selectivity, efficacy, healing time, and three-month scar quality. J Burn Care Res 2017;38(4):e745–55.

14. De Decker I, De Graeve L, Hoeksema H, et al. Enzymatic debridement: past, present, and future. Acta Chir Belg 2022;122(4):279–95.

15. Fouché TW, Bond SM, Vrouwe SQ. Comparing the efficiency of tumescent infiltration techniques in burn surgery. J Burn Care Res 2022;43(3):525–9.

16. Rizzo JA, Ross E, Ostrowski ML, et al. Intraoperative blood transfusions in burn patients. Transfusion 2021;61(Suppl 1):S183–7.

17. Ajai KS, Kumar P, Subair M, et al. Effect of single dose intravenous tranexamic acid on blood loss in tangential excision of burn wounds: a double blind randomised controlled trial. Burns 2022;48(6): 1311–8.

18. Farny B, Fontaine M, Latarjet J, et al. Estimation of blood loss during adult burn surgery. Burns 2018; 44(6):1496–501.

19. Friedstat JS, Klein MB. Acute management of facial burns. Clin Plast Surg 2009;36(4):653–60.

20. MacLennan SE, Wells MD, Neale HW. Reconstruction of the burned breast. Clin Plast Surg 2000; 27(1):113–9.

21. Dantzer E, Queruel P, Salinier L, et al. Dermal regeneration template for deep hand burns: clinical utility for both early grafting and reconstructive surgery. Br J Plast Surg 2003;56(8):764–74.

22. Schulz A, Ribitsch B, Fuchs PC, et al. Treatment of genital burn injuries: traditional procedures and new techniques. Adv Skin Wound Care 2018;31(7): 314–21.

23. Sheridan RL, Greenhalgh D. Special problems in burns. Surg Clin 2014;94(4):781–91.

24. Zajac JC, Liu A, Uselmann AJ, et al. Lighting the way for necrosis excision through indocyanine green fluorescence-guided surgery. J Am Coll Surg 2022; 235(5):743–55.

25. Gupta S, Gupta V, Chanda A. Biomechanical modeling of novel high expansion auxetic skin grafts. Int J Numer Method Biomed Eng 2022; 38(5):e3586.

26. Glaser J, Ziegler B, Hirche C, et al. The status quo of early burn wound excision: insights from the German Burn Registry. Burns 2021;47(6):1259–64.

Skin Substitutes and Autograft Techniques
Temporary and Permanent Coverage Solutions

Elizabeth M. Kenny, MD[a], Tomer Lagziel, MD[b],
C. Scott Hultman, MD, MBA[b,c], Francesco M. Egro, MD, MSc, MRCS[a,d],*

KEYWORDS

• Allograft • Xenograft • Dressings • Skin substitutes • CEA • ReCell • Amnion • Autograft

KEY POINTS

- Autografts remain the gold standard in burn surgery.
- Synthetic dressings, allografts, and xenografts are important options to bridge patients to definitive wound coverage.
- The use of skin substitutes with or without skin grafting is increasingly common especially in highly functional areas.
- Cultured epithelial autograft and ReCell have emerged as strategies to tackle large burn coverage.

INTRODUCTION

Burn injuries are increasingly common, affecting an estimated 2 million people each year worldwide. In the United States alone, 500,000 people undergo medical therapy for their burn injuries, 40,000 patients require hospital admission, and 3000 deaths occur annually.[1] Loss of the protective skin barrier affects temperature regulation, prevention of infection, and evaporative fluid loss. After initial resuscitation, patient stabilization, and debridement of nonviable tissue, attention should be turned to wound coverage as quickly as possible to prevent burn sequela including dehydration, wound infection, sepsis, shock, scarring, and contracture. Coverage of burn injuries remains a challenge to the burn surgeon. Choice of burn coverage depends on a variety of factors:

burn depth, affected surface area, wound bed viability, location, donor site availability, patient comorbidities, cost, and expertise of the reconstructive surgeon. Here, we aim to provide an overview of the temporary and permanent solutions for coverage of burn wounds.

TEMPORARY COVERAGE

The ideal burn dressing exhibits several properties: (1) lack of antigenicity and toxicity, (2) heat and moisture retention, (3) durable barrier to trauma and microorganisms, (4) reduction in pain, (5) ability to adhere and contour to the wound bed, (5) low cost, (6) ease of storage and shelf-life stability, and (7) ability to grow in pediatric patients.[2,3] Although no single dressing exists that exhibits all of these properties, a variety of

[a] Department of Plastic Surgery, University of Pittsburgh Medical Center, Pittsburgh, PA 15261, USA; [b] Department of Plastic and Reconstructive Surgery, The Johns Hopkins University School of Medicine, Baltimore, MD, USA; [c] WPP Plastic and Reconstructive Surgery, WakeMed Health and Hospitals, Raleigh, NC 27610, USA; [d] Department of Surgery, University of Pittsburgh Medical Center, Pittsburgh, PA, USA
* Corresponding author. Department of Plastic Surgery, University of Pittsburgh Medical Center Mercy, 1350 Locust Street, Medical Professional Building, Suite G103, Pittsburgh, PA 15219.
E-mail address: francescoegro@gmail.com

Clin Plastic Surg 51 (2024) 241–254
https://doi.org/10.1016/j.cps.2023.12.001
0094-1298/24/© 2023 Elsevier Inc. All rights reserved.

synthetic and biologic dressings are available for the temporary coverage of superficial or partial-thickness burn wounds.

Synthetic and Biosynthetic Dressings

A variety of dressings have been used in burn management with limited data to suggest superiority of a particular product. The most simplistic of dressings include topical ointments and solutions that can provide a range of antimicrobial and antifungal protection such as bacitracin, polymyxin, nystatin, silver sulfadiazine, mafenide acetate, sodium hypochlorite, silver-containing solutions, and acetic acid (see, Hakan Orbay and colleagues, Prevention and Management of Wound Infections in Burn Patients).[4] Although still essential and effective in burn management to reduce wound infection and promote healing, these therapies are often used as adjuncts to temporary or permanent wound coverage solutions. They do require frequent dressings changes that can cause significant patient discomfort. As such, a variety of synthetic and biosynthetic dressings are now available that can be changed less frequently to alleviate patient discomfort while still protecting against pathogen and fluid loss, providing a moist environment, and promoting reepithelialization and preventing infection. The main advantages of synthetic membranes over biological ones are their constant composition, sterility, and availability. The main disadvantage includes the higher cost. However, a systematic review demonstrated superiority of certain synthetic dressings such as Biobrane in epithelialization rate, length of hospital stay, and pain during treatment.[5] Commonly used synthetic dressings include hydrocolloids, hydrofibers, hydrogels, alginates, and synthetic and biosynthetic membranes as summarized in **Table 1**.[6–13]

Mepilex Ag (Mölnlycke, Göteborg, Sweden, **Fig. 1**) is a soft foam pad that contains silver particles within its structure. The foam pad is coated with a gentle, silicone-based adhesive layer that adheres to the surrounding skin without causing damage on removal. The silver ions are released from the dressing on contact with wound exudate, creating a zone of inhibition. The antimicrobial action of silver helps to reduce the bacterial load and promote a favorable environment for wound healing. The foam pad effectively manages wound exudate with its high absorbency and also helps to maintain a moist wound environment to promote wound healing. The foam is soft, flexible, conformable, and it contours well anywhere in the body. Mepilex Ag is applied to clean debrided burn wounds—most frequently is used for the

treatment of superficial partial-thickness burns. It is left in place for several days and changed in cases of excessive fluid accumulation, worsening of the wound, or signs of infection. Multiple studies have demonstrated the benefit of Mepilex Ag and when compared with other common dressings such as Biobrane, Acticoat, and Aquacel Ag, it achieved faster reepithelialization and better cost effectiveness.[11]

Biobrane (Smith & Nephew, Andover, MA) is a bioengineered skin substitute composed of a silicone layer, which acts as a semipermeable barrier, protecting the wound and reducing pain. The silicone layer is bonded to a nylon mesh, providing structural support and facilitating application and removal. The outer surface is coated with a thin layer of porcine collagen, which promotes wound healing and helps create an optimal environment for tissue regeneration. However, it is prone to infection and reports of toxic shock syndrome have been published. Biobrane is typically applied to debrided burn wounds (most frequently is used for the treatment of superficial partial-thickness burns), and it is generally left in place until the wound has sufficiently healed or until it is ready for definitive wound closure. Biobrane has not been available in the United States since 2016 but remains available around the world.

Acticoat (Smith & Nephew, Andover, MA) is an antimicrobial wound dressing composed of a flexible, low-adherent fabric or foam, coated with a layer of silver nanoparticles. The nanocrystals release silver ions in the presence of wound exudate leading to a localized antimicrobial effect. Acticoat helps to maintain a moist wound environment to promote wound healing and based on the amount of wound exudates the foam can be used for greater absorbency compared with the fabric. Acticoat is applied directly to the partial or full thickness burn wound after appropriate wound cleansing and preparation, and it needs to be changed every 2 to 4 days based on the amount of exudate, or signs of infection.

Aquacel Ag (ConvaTec, Flintshire, UK) is an antimicrobial wound dressing composed of a soft hydrofiber (sodium carboxymethylcellulose fibers) dressing combined with silver ions. When the dressing is exposed to wound exudate, the fibers absorb the fluid and form a gel-like substance, which provides a moist wound environment to support wound healing, helps to minimize trauma during dressing changes, and minimizes the risk of maceration. The silver ions are released from the dressing on contact with wound exudate leading to a localized antimicrobial effect. Aquacel Ag is applied directly to the wounds after appropriate wound cleansing and preparation. Common

Table 1
Common synthetic and biosynthetic burn dressings

Product Name (Company)	Product Description	Advantages	Disadvantages
ABWAT (Aubrey Inc., Carlsbad, CA)[6]	Thin, porous silicone-nylon membrane with embedded porcine type 1 collagen	Ease of application Egress of exudate Adherence to wound bed	Similarities to Biobrane, may have infectious risk (although greater pore size may allow better exudate egress)
Acticoat (Smith & Nephew, Andover, MA)[7]	Trilaminate silver-containing dressing (must be moistened with sterile water to release silver) with a polyethylene net	Antimicrobial	Require frequent dressing changes
Alginates	Absorbent fiber dressing composed of calcium and/or sodium salts	Absorbent Hemostatic	No antimicrobial activity
Aquacel-Ag (ConvaTec, Princeton, NJ)[8]	Aquacel (Hydrofiber dressing of sodium carboxymethylcellulose) impregnated with 1.2% silver	Antimicrobial	Decreased frequency of dressing changes
Biobrane (Dow-Hickham, Sugarland, TX)[9]	Inner layer of nylon mesh (allows fibrovascular ingrowth) and outer silastic layer (barrier to bacteria and moisture retention)	Strong adherence	No antimicrobial activity Infection and TSS risk Not available in the United States
Mepitel (Mölnlycke, Göteborg, Sweden)[10]	Silicone-based nonadhesive net	Allows drainage Ease of change with outer layer dressing	No antimicrobial activity
Mepilex Ag (Mölnlycke, Göteborg, Sweden)[11]	Bilaminar dressing with silver-impregnated polyurethane foam and a silicone-based interface	Antimicrobial silver foam Cost effective Ease of change	Not ideal for highly exudative wounds
PermeaDerm (Milliken Healthcare Products, Portsmouth, NH)[12]	Nylon mesh with silicone. Various iterations that contain collagen or antiscar coatings	Available with various porosity	No antimicrobial activity
TransCyte (Advanced Tissue Sciences, Inc., La Jolla, CA)[13]	Semipermeable silicone membrane and newborn human fibroblast cells on a porcine collagen-coated nylon mesh	Pliable Few dressing changes required	No antimicrobial activity

Abbreviation: TSS, toxic shock syndrome.

indications include partial-thickness burns, donor sites, and chronic wounds. It needs to be changed every 2 to 4 days based on either the amount of exudate or signs of infection.

Alginate dressings (eg, Algisite, Smith & Nephew, Andover, MA; Kaltostat, ConvaTec; Comfeel) are highly absorbent fiber dressing composed of calcium and/or sodium salts of alginic acid, a natural polysaccharide extracted from brown seaweed. The dressing fibers form a gel-like substance when they are exposed to wound exudate, which provides a moist wound environment to support wound healing. Alginates also have inherent hemostatic properties.

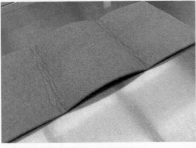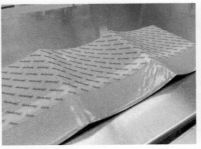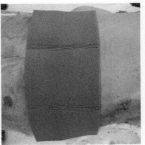

Fig. 1. Mepilex Ag used to treat second-degree burns.

Alginates are often used for donor sites and burn wounds with high volumes of exudates, and they need to be changed every 1 to 3 days based on the amount of exudate.

Biologic Skin Substitutes: Allografts/Xenografts

Many patients who sustain extensive burns are not candidates for autografting due the poor quality of the recipient wound bed and/or to lack of available donor site. In these scenarios, allografting (skin graft from the same species) and xenografting (skin graft from other species) remain viable options to bridge patients to a more definitive reconstruction.

Allografts (Fig. 2) have long remained the temporary burn coverage of choice. They are obtained from cadaveric human skin and can be used in fresh or cryopreserved states. A refrigerated allograft can remain viable up to 2 weeks; however, most recommend cryopreservation of the tissue if not used within a few days of harvest.[14] Once cryopreserved, the allograft can be stored for prolonged periods. The allograft adheres to the

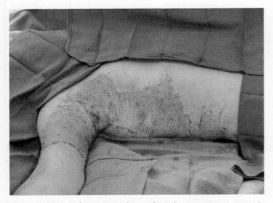

Fig. 2. Allograft to trunk and right upper extremity following excision of mixed second-degree and third-degree burns.

wound bed through a fibrin seal. Fresh allografts undergo vascular ingrowth while frozen allografts do not. An immunocompetent patient will in most cases reject the graft; however, the temporary graft provides a barrier against trauma and fluid loss, reduces pain, and maintains a moist environment for wound bed granulation.[15] Allografts have the benefit of lasting longer than other temporary coverage options, providing durable coverage for up to 3 to 4 weeks depending on the patient's immune response.[16] Although allografting is considered superior to xenografting, supply is more limited and carries the risk of transmission of communicable disease. Allografting is associated with significant cost, particularly with fresh compared with cryopreserved graft.

Compared with allograft, xenografts are less expensive, have longer shelf life, and are more widely available. Similar to allografts, they carry a risk for transmission of communicable disease. Xenografts are ultimately rejected and begin to slough off after approximately 7 days due to immunologic rejection. Despite lack of revascularization, xenografts aid in wound healing by acting as a scaffold for dermal regeneration. They have been associated with reduced pain during dressing changes, protection from physical trauma, antibacterial action, accelerated epidermal growth, and heat and moisture retention.[3] Xenografts have been described from a variety of species including sheep and frog, although porcine dermis and epidermis remains the most widely used xenograft in burn care. Fish-derived skin grafts have been growing in popularity due to shelf stability, low cost, and lack of known transmissible disease, which minimizes processing.[17] Furthermore, there are cultural and religious implications to the use of porcine xenografts. Cold-water species such as the Atlantic cod have higher levels of bioactive lipid mediators. Omega-3 polyunsaturated fatty acids, eicosapentaenoic acid, and docosahexaenoic acid have been shown to aid in wound healing through the modulation of the

Table 2
Common xenograft products for burn coverage

Product Name (Company)	Species	Advantages	Disadvantages
EZ-Derm (Brennen Medical, St. Paul, MN)[21]	Porcine dermis	Lower cost than allograft Aldehyde-treated for better strength and shelf-stable storage	Rejected more quickly than allograft
Kerecis Omega-3 Burn (Kerecis, Reykjavik, Iceland)[22]	Fish skin	Requires minimal processing Shelf-stable	Rejected more quickly than allograft
Mediskin (Brennen Medical, St. Paul, MN)[23]	Porcine skin	Lower cost than allograft	More difficult to store (frozen) Rejected more quickly than allograft

inflammatory process and exhibit antimicrobial properties.[18] Xenograft products can vary in the manner in which they are preserved and sterilized. More recently, xenografts have been modified with techniques such as aldehyde cross-linking and silver ion impregnation to increase antimicrobial action.[19,20] Commonly used commercial products are summarized in **Table 2**.[21–23]

PERMANENT COVERAGE

Temporary burn coverage is crucial in the management of unstable patients or those with extensive injury; however, the ultimate goal is to obtain complete wound coverage as soon as possible with a permanent replacement of the dermal and epidermal skin elements. Permanent coverage of burn wounds can be provided through skin substitutes, autografts (full-thickness grafts [FTSGs] and split-thickness skin grafts [STSG]), and cultured epithelial autografts (CEAs).

Skin Substitutes

Although autologous skin grafting is widely considered the gold standard of burn reconstruction, skin substitutes are commonly required in patients with extensive burn injury that lack sufficient donor site or those with exposure of critical structures such as nerve, vasculature, bone, or tendon. Skin substitutes aim to replace dermis, epidermis, or both skin layers. Skin substitutes can be used as a stand-alone reconstructive option or in conjunction with autologous skin grafting in the reconstruction of deep dermal and full-thickness burn wounds. A variety of skin substitutes are rapidly developing that have historically been categorized as biological or synthetic, although

this differentiation is confounded as human and animal materials are increasingly incorporated into synthetic materials to make composite products. In general, synthetic skin substitutes carry the advantage of the ability to manipulate the scaffold composition while biologic skin substitutes provide a more natural dermis and allow reepithelialization due to the presence of an intact basement membrane. No single product can be labeled the gold standard. Surgeons must weigh a variety of practical factors including product availability, cost, ease of use, storage in selecting the most appropriate skin substitute for their patients. Commonly used synthetic, biologic, and composite skin substitutes are reviewed in **Table 3**.[24–41]

Although uncommonly used in the United States, human amniotic membrane in either fresh or preserved state has commonly been used worldwide for the coverage of superficial burn wounds. Unlike allograft, fetal amnion does not elicit a host immunologic response and is therefore not rejected.[15] Although research in this area is ongoing, there is suggestion that amnion may harbor live stem cells that can accelerate wound healing. Although it functions as a barrier, amnion does so less effectively than epidermal grafts.[42,43] For this reason, some advocate for its use as temporary wound dressing as opposed to a permanent reconstructive option. There is a particular interest in the use of amnion in pediatric patients with burn injuries due to its thinness, pliability, and ease of removal. Although a cost-effective option for superficial burn coverage, limited availability, difficulty in handling, and risk of communicable disease transmission remain barriers to widespread use. Amnion is available in both fresh-

Table 3
Common biologic and synthetic skin substitutes for burn coverage

Product Name (Company)	Product Description	Advantages	Disadvantages
Alloderm (LifeCell Corporation, Branchburg, NJ)[24,25]	Human cadaveric acellularized dermal matrix	Potential for single-stage reconstruction with STSGs Decreased joint contracture	Cost Antigenicity Infection risk Short shelf life
Apligraf (Organogenesis, Inc., Canton, MA)[26]	Bilayered living skin equivalent composed of type I bovine collagen and allogenic keratinocytes and fibroblasts from neonatal foreskin	Can be used for temporary or permanent coverage	Cost Must be applied fresh, short shelf life
Integra (Integra LifeSciences, Princeton, NJ)[27]	Bilayer of decellularized matrix (cross-linked bovine collagen and glycosaminoglycans from shark cartilage) and a semipermeable silicone membrane	Dermal substitute with most published evidence in burn reconstruction	High cost Infection risk
Dermagraft (Advanced BioHealing, LaJolla, CA)[28]	Bioabsorbable polyglactin mesh seeded with allogenic neonatal dermal fibroblasts	Can be used for temporary or permanent coverage Easier to remove than allograft	—
Hyalomatrix (Fidia Advanced Biopolymers, Padua, Italy)[29–31]	Bilayered hyaluronan scaffold with autologous fibroblasts and an outer silicone membrane	Can be used for temporary or permanent coverage	Poorer cosmesis and function when compared with Integra
Matriderm (MedSkin and Health Care AG, Billerbeck, Germany)[32–34]	Single-layer matrix of bovine dermal collagen (I, III, and V) and elastin without cross-linking	Similar results to Integra in animal studies	Infection risk More susceptible to degradation due to no cross-linking
Nevelia (Symatese, Ivry-le-Temple, France)[31,35]	Bilayered porous matrix of bovine type 1 collagen and a semipermeable silicone membrane	Similar results to Integra in animal studies	Limited data in burn population
NovoSorb Biodegradable Temporizing Matrix, BTM (PolyNovo, Melbourne Australia)[36]	Synthetic biodegradable polyurethane dermal matrix with a temporary nonbiodegradable polyurethane seal	Lower cost than Integra an Alloderm Potential for lower infection risk given no biologic material	Limited data in burn population
OASIS (Cook Biotech Inc., West Lafayette, IN)[37]	Extracellular matrix derived from a single layer of porcine small intestinal submucosa	Biologically active ECM	Contraindicated in contaminated wounds Reactions and chronic inflammation are reported

(continued on next page)

Table 3
(continued)

Product Name (Company)	Product Description	Advantages	Disadvantages
OrCel (Fortificell Bioscience, NY)[38]	Bilayered cellular matrix in which allogeneic skin cells (epidermal keratinocytes and dermal fibroblasts from neonatal foreskin) are cultured in 2 layers within a type I bovine collagen sponge	Can be used for temporary coverage or accelerated healing of superficial burn wounds Shelf stable	Allergic reactions are reported
Renoskin (Symatese, Ivry-le-Temple, France)[39]	Bilayered bovine type 1 collagen and silicone membrane	Similar results to Integra in animal studies	Replaced by Nevelia
StrataGraft (StrataTech, A Mallinckrodt Company, Madison, WI)[40,41]	Bilayered murine collagen scaffold with layered allogeneic keratinocytes and dermal fibroblasts	Can reduce or eliminate the need for autograft	Pruritis Blistering Hypertrophic scar

frozen and glycerol-preserved forms. The most commonly used products are seen in **Table 4** and **Fig. 3**.[44,45]

Autografts

Skin grafting remains at the core of burn reconstruction. When performing an autograft, the surgeon must consider graft thickness and whether meshing is required. FTSGs are composed of the entire epidermis and dermis, whereas STSGs contain the epidermis and superficial portion of dermis. FTSGs provide a cosmetically superior result due to better color match, presence of adnexal structures, and lower likelihood of contracture; however, the use of FTSG is often limited to facial reconstruction and coverage over joint surfaces due to limited donor site availability, need to close the donor site primarily, and higher likelihood of graft failure. FTSG are more often used in secondary burn reconstruction than during acute burn care.

Table 4
Common amnion products for burn coverage

Product Name (Company)	Product Description	Advantages	Disadvantages
Acelagraft; Celgene Cellular Therapeutics, Cedar Knolls, NJ)	Decellularized and dehydrated human amnionic membrane	Shelf stable	Limited data in burn literature
Amniofill (MiMedx, Marietta, GA)	Placental extracellular matrix	Structural integrity	Limited data in burn literature
AmnioGraft and Amnioguard (BioTissue, Doral, FL)	Cryopreserved amnion	Variable thicknesses available	Most data in ocular injury Storage (frozen)
EpiFix and EpiBurn (MiMedx Group Inc., Marietta, GA)[44]	Dehydrated human amnion/chorion membranes	Shelf stable	Loss of structural integrity
Grafix (Osiris Therapeutics, Inc., Columbia, MD)[45]	Cryopreserved placental membrane	Maintained structural and cellular integrity	Storage (fresh frozen)

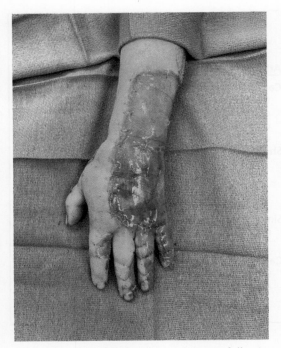

Fig. 3. Integra to left hand and forearm following excision of mixed second-degree and third-degree burns.

Although STSGs are often more painful for patients and result in poorer cosmesis and higher risk of contracture, they have a lower likelihood of graft failure compared with FTSGs. Furthermore, STSG donor sites are more readily available, can be used for repeat harvests, and do not require closure. The depth of an STSG can generally vary from 0.008 to 0.020 inches based on recipient site and age of the patients. Thicker grafts carry lower rates of contracture and improved cosmesis at the risk of poorer graft take. If the decision is made to proceed with split-thickness skin grafting, the surgeon must also decide whether to use meshed versus sheet grafts. STSGs are commonly meshed anywhere from 1.5:1 to 6:1 in the burn population. Although meshing of skin grafts can allow coverage of large surface areas while limiting the size of the required donor sites, the fenestrated appearance of meshed grafts is difficult to eliminate (**Fig. 4**). Meshed grafts are prone to hypertrophic scarring due to the healing by secondary intention that occurs in the interstices. For patients with extensive burn surface area, widely meshed grafts (6:1 mesh ratio or greater) may be required. Widely meshed grafts have a high risk of graft loss but studies suggest that placing an allograft overlay can allow for graft take at up to a 9:1 mesh ratio as described in the Meeks or sandwich technique.[46]

Cultured Epithelial Autografts and Spray Techniques

CEA is a relatively new advancement in burn care, with the first clinical description for its use in full-thickness burns described in 1981.[47] Using ex vivo cellular expansion, autologous keratinocytes from a small skin biopsy can be used to cover a large surface area. Expansion typically takes 2 to 5 weeks, and cells can be applied in confluent sheets as well as spray-on suspensions. With advances in critical care medicine, patients sustaining burns exceeding 90% or more of total body surface area can survive their trauma.[48] For these patients, CEA may be the only option for autologous reconstruction. Data on the efficacy of CEA remains mixed.[49] There is growing evidence that CEA in combination with STSGs is superior to either treatment alone.[50] The high cost of CEA, fragility of grafts, lack of dermal substitute, time required to culture the keratinocytes, and variable results regarding take and durability remain a barrier to widespread use of this technique in burn management. Commonly used CEA products and spray techniques can be seen in **Table 5** and **Fig. 5**.[51–57]

The Johns Hopkins Burn Surgery group performed a retrospective cohort study of 52 burn patients who were treated with CEA between January 1, 1988, and December 31, 2021. Patients were divided into predefined groups: Group 1 (early era: 1988–1999) = 11 patients, Group 2 (premodern era: 2000–2010) = 10 patients, and Group 3 (Modern era: 2011–2021) = 31 patients. The mean percentage total burn surface area (% TBSA) values were 70% in the early era, 68% in the premodern era, and 63% in the modern era. All demographics were comparable among the groups. **Table 6** shows all demographic data.

The study showed lower mortality rates in the early and modern era groups (Group 1 = 20%, Group 2 = 60%, and Group 3 = 27%, $P < .05$), although the predicted mortality based on revised Baux Scores was not significantly different between the groups (Group 1 = 53%, Group 2 = 47%, and Group 3 = 49%, NS). Patients in the early era group also had an overall shorter hospital length of stay (Group 1 = 90 days, Group 2 = 127 days, and Group 3 = 205 days, $P < .05$). Finally, the surface area grafted per patient was the highest in the modern era group (Group 1 = 2000 cm^2, Group 2 = 4187 cm^2, and Group 3 = 4090 cm^2, $P < .05$). The differences in complication rates among the 3 groups were not statistically significant. The results are shown in **Fig. 6** and **Tables 7** and **8**.

ReCell (Avita Medical, Inc., Valencia, CA) is a newer technology provided as a single-use kit for

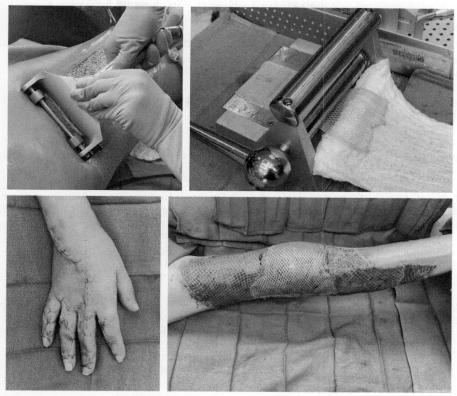

Fig. 4. Split-thickness skin graft. Top left, harvesting using an air dermatome; Top right, STSG being meshed 2:1 ratio; Bottom left, pie crusted sheet of STSG; Bottom right, STSG meshed 3:1 ratio (thigh and lower leg) and 2:1 ratio (knee).

extraction and application of aerosolized, noncultured epidermal cells. ReCell has several advantages when compared with other CEA products: (1) the ReCell suspension includes all epidermal cells (keratinocytes, melanocytes, fibroblasts, and Langerhans cells) rather than keratinocyte-only products; (2) ReCell has been demonstrated to have an 80:1 expansion ratio where 1 mL of suspension is generated from 1 cm^2 of donor site and can be applied for coverage of an 80 cm^2 wound; and (3) ReCell is prepared intraoperatively without off-site culturing, eliminating the need for weeks of cell expansion between harvest and application. ReCell was approved for use in burn reconstruction by the Food and Drug Administration in 2018 following a series of studies that showed similar outcomes between ReCell and STSGs in terms of wound closure, pain, and scarring.[56,58,59] Compared with patients who underwent split-thickness skin grafting, patients who were treated with ReCell experienced significantly less donor site pain, faster rates of donor site healing, approximately 40 times smaller donor sites, and higher patient satisfaction. It is currently being used in burn centers across the nation.[60,61]

Flaps, Tissue Expansion, and Microsurgical Reconstruction

Although beyond the scope of this article, other forms of autologous reconstruction play a crucial role in burn care. Locoregional flaps, tissue expansion, and microsurgical free flap reconstruction are considered for acute burn reconstruction when more durable coverage of vital structures such as nerve, vasculature, tendon, or bone is needed. More commonly, these techniques are used in delayed burn reconstruction to manage esthetic or functional concerns from scarring and contracture. Algorithms and considerations for more advanced reconstructive techniques have been reviewed extensively elsewhere.[62–65]

FUTURE DIRECTIONS

Because survival rates after burn injuries continue to increase, attention in burn care is shifting to

Table 5
Common cultured epithelial autograft products and spray techniques for burn coverage

Product Name (Company)	Product Description	Advantages	Disadvantages
CellSpray XP (Clinical Cell Culture Ltd [C3])[51]	Noncultured spray suspension of keratinocytes	Faster to use than cultured products	Requires 2 d of processing
Epicel (Vericel, Cambridge, MA)[52]	Sheets of cultured keratinocytes	2–8 cell layers thick	Blistering Pruritis Squamous cell carcinoma risk
JACE (Japan Tissue Engineering Co., Ltd. Japan)[53]	Sheets of cultured keratinocytes	Similar to Epicel	Similar to Epicel
Keraheal (Biosolution Co. Ltd, Seoul, Korea)[54]	Spray suspension of epidermal cells	Shorter culturing time than sheets Full complement of epidermal cells	Requires culture
MySkin (Regenerys, Cambridge, UK)[55]	Sheets of keratinocytes on silicone with plasma polymer	Similar to Epicel Inclusion of plasma may promote healing	Limited data
ReCell (Ativa Medical, Valencia, CA)[56]	Spray suspension of epidermal cells	Prepared intraoperatively with no need for off-site culturing Full complement of epidermal cells	No dermal component
SkinGun and CellMist (RenovaCare, Inc., NY)[57]	Spray suspension of epidermal and stem cells	Stem cells offer regenerative therapy Prepared intraoperatively with no need for off-site culturing Full complement of epidermal cells	Limited data

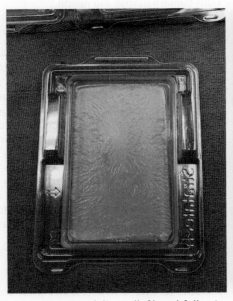 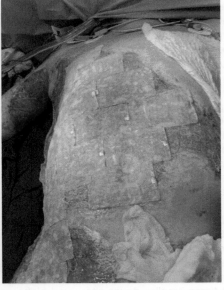

Fig. 5. CEA appearance on delivery (*left*) and following application on a third-degree burn of the trunk.

Table 6
Patient demographics receiving cultured epithelial autograft

	Group 1 (n = 31) 1988–1999	Group 2 (n = 10) 2000–2010	Group 3 (n = 11) 2011–Present	P-Value
Age (y)	33.62 ± 7.03	36.95 ± 14.20	36.46 ± 14.19	NS
Sex	M = 87% F = 13%	M = 90% F = 10%	M = 64% F = 36%	NS —
%TBSA	69.77 ± 7.40	67.76 ± 17.20	63.27 ± 22.54	NS
%TBSA range	50–91	35–96	43–90	—
Inhalation injury (%)	70.97	31.58	45.46	NS

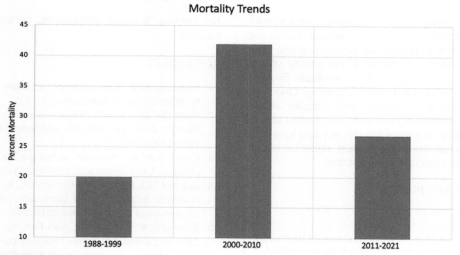

Fig. 6. Mortality trends over time.

optimization of patient function and cosmesis. Although advances have been made in restoration of dermal and epidermal structures, no current skin substitutes restore adnexal structures. Research continues into bioengineered skin substitutes that contain all skin components and cell types.[66] Furthermore, many products can only replicate either the dermal or epidermal elements, although new products such as cell-seeded scaffolds are emerging that mimic full-thickness skin. Another area that remains promising is the potential for 3-dimensional bioprinting.[67] This technique would allow layered deposition of cells along scaffolding materials to quickly and reproducibly fabricate skin substitutes.

Table 7
Outcomes measured

	Group 1 (n = 31) 1988–1999	Group 2 (n = 10) 2000–2010	Group 3 (n = 11) 2011–Present	P-Value
Hospital LOS (d)	89.73 ± 23.69	126.5 ± 139.22	205.09 ± 168.30	<.05*
Complications (%)	55	90	64	NS
Mean graft coverage (cm²)	2006.67 ± 587.19	4187.14 ± 1696.43	4090.00 ± 1280.46	<.01*
Mortality (%)	20	60	27	<.05*

Table 2. Outcomes measured.
*p<0.05 is statistically significant.

Table 8
Predicted v. actual mortality

	Revised Baux Score	Predicted Mortality (%)	Actual Mortality (%)	P-Value[a]
Group 1 (n = 31) 1988–1999	115.45 +/8.69	49.53	20	<.05*
Group 2 (n = 10) 2000–2010	1 13.30 ± 19.86	47.11	42	NS
Group 3 (n = 11) 2011–present	107.45 ± 31.57	48.89	27	<.01*

[a] P-value indicated statistical significance between predicted and actual mortality.

SUMMARY

Prompt coverage of burn wounds is vital to minimize infection and improve patient outcomes. Although the principles of burn coverage have largely remained unchanged, the variety of synthetic and biological products available to assist the burn surgeon is rapidly changing. One must be prepared to constantly and critically assess the data on emerging products, and further studies are needed to compare the efficacy and long-term outcomes of the various skin substitutes and autologous reconstructive options.

CLINICS CARE POINTS

- Coverage of burn wounds is crucial to prevent sequalae including dehydration, wound infection, sepsis, shock, scarring, and contracture.

- Numerous temporary and permanent options for coverage of burn wounds have been described.

- Temporary options for burn coverage include synthetic dressings, allografts, and xenografts. These are important options to bridge patients to definitive wound coverage.

- Permanent burn coverage can be achieved through skin substitutes, CEA, ReCell, amnion, and autografting.

- Autografts remain the gold standard in burn surgery.

- The use of skin substitutes with or without skin grafting is increasingly common especially in highly functional areas.

- CEA and ReCell have emerged as strategies to tackle large burn coverage.

ACKNOWLEDGMENTS

No Acknowledgments.

DISCLOSURES

No funding, financial disclosures, or sources of support.

REFERENCES

1. Association AB. Burn incidence fact sheet. Chicago, IL: American Burn Association; 2019.
2. Pruitt BA, Levine NS. Characteristics and uses of biologic dressings and skin substitutes. Arch Surg 1984;119(3):312–22.
3. Chiu T, Burd A. "Xenograft" dressing in the treatment of burns. Clin Dermatol 2005;23(4):419–23.
4. Jeschke MG, Shahrokhi S, Finnerty CC, et al. Wound coverage technologies in burn care: established techniques. J Burn Care Res 2018;39(3):313–8.
5. Vloemans A, Hermans M, Van Der Wal M, et al. Optimal treatment of partial thickness burns in children: a systematic review. Burns 2014;40(2):177–90.
6. Vandenberg VB. AWBATTM: early clinical experience. Eplasty 2010;10.
7. Wasiak J, Cleland H, Campbell F, et al. Dressings for superficial and partial thickness burns. Cochrane Database Syst Rev 2013;(3).
8. Verbelen J, Hoeksema H, Heyneman A, et al. Aquacel® Ag dressing versus Acticoat™ dressing in partial thickness burns: a prospective, randomized, controlled study in 100 patients. Part 1: burn wound healing. Burns 2014;40(3):416–27.
9. Whitaker IS, Prowse S, Potokar TS. A critical evaluation of the use of Biobrane as a biologic skin substitute: a versatile tool for the plastic and reconstructive surgeon. Ann Plast Surg 2008;60(3): 333–7.
10. Gee Kee E, Kimble RM, Cuttle L, et al. Comparison of three different dressings for partial thickness burns in children: study protocol for a randomised controlled trial. Trials 2013;14:1–8.
11. Aggarwala S, Harish V, Roberts S, et al. Treatment of partial thickness burns: a prospective, randomized controlled trial comparing four routinely used burns dressings in an ambulatory care setting. J Burn Care Res 2021;42(5):934–43.

12. Woodroof A, Phipps R, Woeller C, et al. Evolution of a biosynthetic temporary skin substitute: a preliminary study. Eplasty 2015;15.

13. Demling R, DeSanti L. Closure of partial-thickness facial burns with a bioactive skin substitute in the major burn population decreases the cost of care and improves outcome. Wounds-A Compendium of Clinical Research And Practice 2002;14(6):230–4.

14. Robb EC, Bechmann N, Plessinger RT, et al. Storage media and temperature maintain normal anatomy of cadaveric human skin for transplantation to full-thickness skin wounds. J Burn Care Rehabil 2001; 22(6):393–6.

15. Palackic A, Duggan RP, Campbell MS, et al. The role of skin substitutes in acute burn and reconstructive burn surgery: an updated comprehensive review. Paper presented at: Seminars in Plastic Surgery 2022.

16. Saffle JR. Closure of the excised burn wound: temporary skin substitutes. Clin Plast Surg 2009;36(4): 627–41.

17. Luze H, Nischwitz SP, Smolle C, et al. The use of acellular fish skin grafts in burn wound management—a systematic review. Medicina 2022;58(7): 912.

18. Alam K, Jeffery SL. Acellular fish skin grafts for management of split thickness donor sites and partial thickness burns: a case series. Mil Med 2019; 184(Supplement_1):16–20.

19. Shores JT, Gabriel A, Gupta S. Skin substitutes and alternatives: a review. Adv Skin Wound Care 2007; 20(9):493–508.

20. Halim AS, Khoo TL, Yussof SJM. Biologic and synthetic skin substitutes: an overview. Indian J Plast Surg 2010;43(S 01):S23–8.

21. Troy J, Karlnoski R, Downes K, et al. The use of EZ Derm® in partial-thickness burns: an institutional review of 157 patients. Eplasty 2013;13.

22. Kim YJ, Wood SM, Yoon AP, et al. Efficacy of nonoperative treatments for lateral epicondylitis: a systematic review and meta-analysis. Plast Reconstr Surg 2021;147(1):112–25.

23. Karlsson M, Lindgren M, Jarnhed-Andersson I, et al. Dressing the split-thickness skin graft donor site: a randomized clinical trial. Adv Skin Wound Care 2014;27(1):20–5.

24. Callcut R, Schurr M, Sloan M, et al. Clinical experience with Alloderm: a one-staged composite dermal/epidermal replacement utilizing processed cadaver dermis and thin autografts. Burns 2006; 32(5):583–8.

25. Yim H, Cho YS, Seo CH, et al. The use of AlloDerm on major burn patients: AlloDerm prevents post-burn joint contracture. Burns 2010;36(3):322–8.

26. Waymack P, Duff RG, Sabolinski M, et al. The effect of a tissue engineered bilayered living skin analog, over meshed split-thickness autografts on the healing of excised burn wounds. Burns 2000;26(7): 609–19.

27. Dantzer E, Braye FM. Reconstructive surgery using an artificial dermis (Integra): results with 39 grafts. Br J Plast Surg 2001;54(8):659–64.

28. Purdue GF, Hunt JL, Still JM Jr, et al. A multicenter clinical trial of a biosynthetic skin replacement, Dermagraft-TC, compared with cryopreserved human cadaver skin for temporary coverage of excised burn wounds. J Burn Care Rehabil 1997; 18(1):52–7.

29. Erbatur S, Coban YK, Aydın EN. Comparision of clinical and histopathological results of hyalomatrix usage in adult patients. International journal of burns and trauma 2012;2(2):118.

30. Gravante G, Sorge R, Merone A, et al. Hyalomatrix PA in burn care practice: results from a national retrospective survey, 2005 to 2006. Ann Plast Surg 2010;64(1):69–79.

31. Nicoletti G, Tresoldi MM, Malovini A, et al. Versatile use of dermal substitutes: a retrospective survey of 127 consecutive cases. Indian J Plast Surg 2018; 51(01):046–53.

32. Bloemen MC, van Leeuwen MC, van Vucht NE, et al. Dermal substitution in acute burns and reconstructive surgery: a 12-year follow-up. Plast Reconstr Surg 2010;125(5):1450–9.

33. Schneider J, Biedermann T, Widmer D, et al. Matriderm® versus Integra®: a comparative experimental study. Burns 2009;35(1):51–7.

34. Dickson K, Lee KC, Abdulsalam A, et al. A histological and clinical study of MatriDerm® use in burn reconstruction. J Burn Care Res 2023;2(1). irad024.

35. Yiğitbaş H, Yavuz E, Beken Özdemir E, et al. Our experience with dermal substitute Nevelia® in the treatment of severely burned patients. Ulus Travma Acil Cerrahi Derg 2019;25(5):520–6.

36. Greenwood JE, Schmitt BJ, Wagstaff MJ. Experience with a synthetic bilayer biodegradable temporising matrix in significant burn injury. Burns Open 2018;2(1):17–34.

37. Shi L, Ronfard V. Biochemical and biomechanical characterization of porcine small intestinal submucosa (SIS): a mini review. International journal of burns and trauma 2013;3(4):173.

38. Still J, Glat P, Silverstein P, et al. The use of a collagen sponge/living cell composite material to treat donor sites in burn patients. Burns 2003; 29(8):837–41.

39. Philandrianos C, Andrac-Meyer L, Mordon S, et al. Comparison of five dermal substitutes in full-thickness skin wound healing in a porcine model. Burns 2012;38(6):820–9.

40. Gibson AL, Holmes IVJH, Shupp JW, et al. A phase 3, open-label, controlled, randomized, multicenter trial evaluating the efficacy and safety of

StrataGraft® construct in patients with deep partial-thickness thermal burns. Burns 2021;47(5):1024–37.

41. Holmes IVJH, Cancio LC, Carter JE, et al. Pooled safety analysis of STRATA2011 and STRATA2016 clinical trials evaluating the use of StrataGraft® in patients with deep partial-thickness thermal burns. Burns 2022;48(8):1816–24.

42. Yang C, Xiong AB, He XC, et al. Efficacy and feasibility of amniotic membrane for the treatment of burn wounds: a meta-analysis. J Trauma Acute Care Surg 2021;90(4):744–55.

43. Kesting MR, Wolff K-D, Hohlweg-Majert B, et al. The role of allogenic amniotic membrane in burn treatment. J Burn Care Res 2008;29(6):907–16.

44. Dai C, Shih S, Khachemoune A. Skin substitutes for acute and chronic wound healing: an updated review. J Dermatol Treat 2020;31(6):639–48.

45. Johnson EL, Tassis EK, Michael GM, et al. Viable placental allograft as a biological dressing in the clinical management of full-thickness thermal occupational burns: two case reports. Medicine 2017; 96(49).

46. Kreis R, Mackie D, Hermans R, et al. Expansion techniques for skin grafts: comparison between mesh and Meek island (sandwich-) grafts. Burns 1994;20:S39–42.

47. O'Connor N, Mulliken J, Banks-Schlegel S, et al. Grafting of burns with cultured epithelium prepared from autologous epidermal cells. Lancet 1981; 317(8211):75–8.

48. AlAlwan MA, Almomin HA, Shringarpure SD, et al. Survival from ninety-five percent total body surface area burn: a case report and literature review. Cureus 2022;14(2).

49. Wood F, Kolybaba M, Allen P. The use of cultured epithelial autograft in the treatment of major burn injuries: a critical review of the literature. Burns 2006; 32(4):395–401.

50. Chrapusta A, Nessler MB, Drukala J, et al. A comparative analysis of advanced techniques for skin reconstruction with autologous keratinocyte culture in severely burned children: own experience. Advances in Dermatology and Allergology/Postępy Dermatologii i Alergologii 2014;31(3):164–9.

51. Zweifel C, Contaldo C, Köhler C, et al. Initial experiences using non-cultured autologous keratinocyte suspension for burn wound closure. J Plast Reconstr Aesthetic Surg 2008;61(11):e1–4.

52. Domaszewska-Szostek AP, Krzyżanowska MO, Czarnecka AM, et al. Local treatment of burns with cell-based therapies tested in clinical studies. J Clin Med 2021;10(3):396.

53. Matsumura H, Matsushima A, Ueyama M, et al. Application of the cultured epidermal autograft "JACE®" for treatment of severe burns: results of a 6-year multicenter surveillance in Japan. Burns 2016;42(4):769–76.

54. Yim H, Yang HT, Cho YS, et al. Clinical study of cultured epithelial autografts in liquid suspension in severe burn patients. Burns 2011;37(6):1067–71.

55. Moustafa M, Bullock AJ, Creagh FM, et al. Randomized, controlled, single-blind study on use of autologous keratinocytes on a transfer dressing to treat nonhealing diabetic ulcers. Regen Med 2007;Nov; 2(6):887–902. https://doi.org/10.2217/17460751.2.6.887. PMID: 18034628.

56. Holmes Iv JH, Molnar JA, Carter JE, et al. A comparative study of the ReCell® device and autologous split-thickness meshed skin graft in the treatment of acute burn injuries. J Burn Care Res 2018;39(5):694–702.

57. Gerlach JC, Johnen C, McCoy E, et al. Autologous skin cell spray-transplantation for a deep dermal burn patient in an ambulant treatment room setting. Burns 2011;37(4):e19–23.

58. Holmes IVJ, Molnar J, Shupp J, et al. Demonstration of the safety and effectiveness of the RECELL® System combined with split-thickness meshed autografts for the reduction of donor skin to treat mixed-depth burn injuries. Burns 2019;45(4): 772–82.

59. Sood R, Roggy DE, Zieger MJ, et al. A comparative study of spray keratinocytes and autologous meshed split-thickness skin graft in the treatment of acute burn injuries. Wounds: a compendium of clinical research and practice 2015;27(2):31–40.

60. Ozhathil DK, Tay MW, Wolf SE, et al. A narrative review of the history of skin grafting in burn care. Medicina 2021;57(4):380.

61. Holmes IVJH. A brief history of RECELL® and its current indications. J Burn Care Res 2023; 44(Supplement_1):S48–9.

62. Hespe GE, Burns Levi B. Acute care and reconstruction. In: Plastic surgery-principles and practice. Elsevier; 2022. p. 155–71.

63. Ibrahim A, Skoracki R, Goverman J, et al. Microsurgery in the burn population–a review of the literature. Annals of Burns and Fire Disasters 2015;28(1):39.

64. Alessandri Bonetti M, Jeong T, Stofman GM, Egro FM. A 10-Year Single-Burn Center Review of Free Tissue Transfer for Burn-Related Injuries. J Burn Care Res 2024 Jan 5;45(1):130–5. https://doi.org/10.1093/jbcr/irad132. PMID: 37703393.

65. Kasmirski JA, Alessandri-Bonetti M, Liu H, et al. Free flap failure and complications in acute burns: a systematic review and meta-analysis. Plastic and Reconstructive Surgery–Global Open 2023;11(10):e5311.

66. Takami Y, Yamaguchi R, Ono S, et al. Clinical application and histological properties of autologous tissue-engineered skin equivalents using an acellular dermal matrix. J Nippon Med Sch 2014;81(6): 356–63.

67. Varkey M, Visscher DO, Van Zuijlen PP, et al. Skin bioprinting: the future of burn wound reconstruction? Burns & trauma 2019;7.

Prevention and Management of Wound Infections in Burn Patients

Hakan Orbay, MD, PhD[a], Jenny A. Ziembicki, MD[b],
Mohamed Yassin, MD, PhD, MBA[c], Francesco M. Egro, MD, MSc, MRCS[a,b,*]

KEYWORDS

- Burns • Infections • Wound infections • Prevention • Treatment • Management

KEY POINTS

- Burn wounds are at increased risk of infection due to loss of skin barrier and general immune compromised status of burn patients.
- Most common bacteria causing burn wound infections are *Staphylococcus aureus* and *Pseudomonas aeruginosa*. Multidrug resistance is common in burn wound infections.
- Untreated infections can result in sepsis and septic shock, which is the most common cause of mortality in burn patients.
- Preventive efforts should be maximized via the use of infection control preventive measures, regular change of lines, topical antimicrobials, and adequate surgical intervention.

BACKGROUND

According to the United States National Burn Repository, the main source of morbidity in burn patients has shifted during the last decade from anoxic injury to infection and sepsis.[1,2] The most common infectious etiologies are pneumonia, urinary tract infection, cellulitis, and wound infection. According to recent literature, 42% to 65% of burn-related deaths during the past decade were attributable to infectious complications.[3–6] These infections could be bacterial, viral, or fungal.[7]

Burn injury initiates a complex physiologic response resulting in immunosuppression and vulnerability to nosocomial bacterial infections.[7,8] With the loss of the skin barrier and accumulation of biological fluids, also known as burn wound exudates, burn wounds turn into a niche environment for infections.[9,10] Additionally, necrotic eschar tissue over the burn wounds provides a favorable protein-rich platform for microbial biofilm formation[11–13] and releases toxins, which further impairs local host immune responses.[14–17] Liberal use of antibiotics in this setting does not prevent infections; on the contrary, it contributes to the increase of multidrug-resistant (MDR) organisms.[18–20]

BURN WOUND COLONIZATION AND BIOFILM FORMATION

The primary source of colonization for burn wounds is the environment and the patients' gut and nasopharyngeal tracts. Per American Burn Association (ABA) Consensus Conference in 2007, wound colonization is described as low concentration of bacteria on the wound surface, absence of invasive infection, and less than 10^5 bacteria per gram of tissue.[15]

[a] Department of Plastic Surgery, University of Pittsburgh Medical Center, Pittsburgh, PA, USA; [b] Department of Surgery, University of Pittsburgh Medical Center, Pittsburgh, PA; [c] Division of Infectious Diseases, University of Pittsburgh Medical Center, Pittsburgh, PA, USA
* Corresponding author. Department of Plastic Surgery, University of Pittsburgh Medical Center, 1350 Locust Street, Medical Professional Building, Suite G103, Pittsburgh, PA 15219.
E-mail address: francescoegro@gmail.com

Clin Plastic Surg 51 (2024) 255–265
https://doi.org/10.1016/j.cps.2023.11.003
0094-1298/24/© 2023 Elsevier Inc. All rights reserved.

plasticsurgery.theclinics.com

Burn wounds are initially colonized by gram-positive organisms, consistent with the normal resident flora of the skin but over time gram-negative organisms begin to colonize the wound as well. *Pseudomonas aeruginosa* is the most common gram-negative organism that colonizes burn wounds.[21,22] Unfortunately, MDR is very common among *Pseudomonas* organisms.[1] The mean number of days from admission to identification of *Pseudomonas* in burn wounds can be as low as 10 days.[2] Methicillin-resistant *Staphylococcus aureus* (MRSA) can colonize the burn wounds early during hospitalization if the patients are nasal carriers.[11] *Acinetobacter calcoaceticus-baumannii* is another common MDR gram-negative nosocomial organism that colonizes burn wounds.[11,21,22]

Biofilm formed by these bacteria allows them to escape the host immune response.[23,24] Reversible attachment of these bacteria to the wound surface is the first step of biofilm formation followed by irreversible attachment and production of extracellular matrix. The biofilm matures as the bacteria encase themselves within this matrix. A mature biofilm can release aggregates of bacteria infecting new sites within the wound[25,26] (**Fig. 1**). Bacteria growing in a biofilm are 10 and 1000 times more resistant to antibiotics compared with planktonic bacteria.[27] As a result, they are difficult to eradicate.[6] In addition to becoming a continuous source of infection, biofilm formation also arrests the wounds in the inflammation stage.[28,29] Accumulation of immune cells at the wound site, in response to biofilm, creates a persistent inflammatory state delaying reepithelization and closure of the wound.[30]

BURN WOUND INFECTION

Distinguishing between burn wound infection and colonization can be challenging.[31] Physical examination of the patient is crucial to assist in obtaining the correct diagnosis. Burn wound erythema is a physiologic phenomenon produced by inflammatory mediators from tissues surrounding the burn area. This differs by true burn wound infection by the milder form of erythema that is local and not spreading, as well as the absence of purulent discharge or wound necrosis. Normally, the erythema presents early on (within first few days of burn injury) and lasts approximately 1 week. Burn cellulitis is a soft tissue noninvasive infection leading to erythema surrounding the wound and worsening with time, edema, induration, pain, wound discharge or purulence, and possible ascending lymphangitis. Systemic symptoms may also be present such as fever, nausea, vomiting, chills,

and leukocytosis. Colonization is common in critically ill patients, particularly in patients requiring prolonged mechanical ventilation.[32] Definitive diagnosis of infection can be established with quantitative analysis of tissue cultures (pathogen count) and histologic examination.[15,31] The traditional definition of invasive infection includes bacterial counts exceeding 10^5 organisms per gram of tissue.[33] If burn wound colony counts from biopsies or after cleaning of the surface of the wound are greater than 10^5 per gram of tissue, the graft survival rate is only 19%, compared with 94% chance of graft survival if colony counts are less than 10^5 per gram of tissue.[34] However, qualitative (pathogen detected or not detected) or semiquantitative (grading of pathogen presence in wound as scant, few, moderate, or heavy) tests largely replaced histologic diagnosis of burn infections due to increased labor and cost associated with the latter.[15] The authors believe that the best way to diagnose wound infection is based on a combination of microbiologic and histologic specimens. Microbiology data are more sensitive and will determine the presence of bacteria in a semiquantitative fashion, whereas histology will determine the depth of infection and provide a better idea of the extent of the infection by finding bacteria or fungi deeper in the tissues with signs of lymphocytic infiltration and vascular invasion.

A variety of bacterial, viral, and fungal pathogens can lead to burn wound infections and a summary of the microorganisms can be found in **Table 1**.[15] MRSA and *Enterococcus* species (ie, *Enterococcus faecalis*) are the most common gram-positive bacteria isolated from burn wound infections,[16,21,35] whereas *P aeruginosa* and *Klebsiella pneumoniae* constitute the most common gram-negative microorganisms.[36] Bacterial infections in burn patients could result in multiple cases or isolated cases. Infections in burn patients are particularly susceptible to cause outbreaks.

Viral infections occurring in burn patients include a long list of viruses. Immunocompromised state in burn patients may also allow reactivation of latent infections caused by herpes simplex virus (HSV), cytomegalovirus (CMV), and varicella zoster virus. Additionally, burn victims are particularly susceptible to respiratory viral infections including coronavirus disease 2019, influenza, and respiratory syncytial viruses. These viral infections increase morbidity and mortality in severely burned patients.[17] Most of these infections are systemic and not necessarily limited to the skin.

Burn patients are also prone to invasive fungal infections caused by opportunistic fungi (**Fig. 2**). Most modern burn centers are equipped with temperature and moisture-regulated patient rooms.

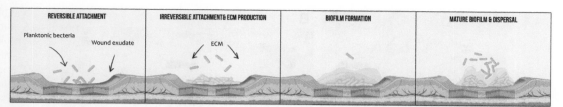

Fig. 1. The stages of biofilm formation in burn wounds. (*Adapted from* Maslova E, Eisaiankhongi L, Sjöberg F, McCarthy RR. Burns and biofilms: priority pathogens and in vivo models. NPJ Biofilms Microbiomes. 2021;7(1):73. Published 2021 Sep 9.)

The air in these rooms is exchanged rapidly through microbial filters to prevent the spread of fungal spores.[37] In patients with large burns, additional external heating measures may be used to provide normothermia. Despite the benefits in terms of wound healing and physiologic resuscitation, the combination of external heat, moisturized wound dressings, compromised immunity, and the lack of epidermal barrier provides a milieu that increases the risk of fungal colonization and infection.[38] The most common fungus causing infection in burn patients is *Candida albicans* (85%).[39–42] Nevertheless, there is an increasing incidence of invasive fungal infections caused by non-albicans *Candida*, *Aspergillus*, and Zygomycetes including *Mucor* spp.[33,41] These infections are a significant cause of late-onset morbidity and mortality in patients with large burns.[15] The risk of infection is correlated directly with burned total body surface area (TBSA), inhalational lung injury, and comorbidities such as increased age, uncontrolled diabetes, and the presence of central venous catheters[38,40,43,44] **(Box 1)**. The overall incidence of fungal contamination and infection in burn patients ranges between 6.3% and 15%.[45,46] It should be noted that the incidence of fungal infections in patients presenting with greater than 80% TBSA may be lower because of early demise of these patients before the development of fungal infections.[15] Diagnosis of fungal infections remains to be challenging. Direct confirmation of positive fungal cultures from burn wounds is the gold standard for diagnosis but requires a long time and may delay the treatment.[47,48]

Table 1
Pathogens causing burn wound infection

Group	Species
Gram-positive organisms	*S aureus* MRSA Coagulase-negative staphylococci *Enterococcus* spp Vancomycin-resistant enterococci
Gram-negative organisms	*P aeruginosa* *Escherichia coli* *K pneumoniae* *Serratia marcescens* *Enterobacter* spp *Proteus* spp *Acinetobacter* spp *Bacteroides* spp
Fungi	*Candida* spp *Aspergillus* spp *Fusarium* spp *Alternaria* spp *Rhizopus* spp *Mucor* spp
Viruses	HSV CMV Varicella-zoster virus

Adapted from Church D, Elsayed S, Reid O, Winston B, Lindsay R. Burn wound infections. Clin Microbiol Rev. 2006;19(2):403-434.

CHONDRITIS

Aside from soft tissue infections, infections involving cartilage are often seen in patients with burn wounds in the ears. Skin overlying the pinna is thin and underlying cartilage gets easily exposed in case of a burn injury. Exposed cartilage is at risk for infection. Typical clinical signs of chondritis are edema of the ear that causes protrusion of the pinna from the head and tenderness to palpation. Mafenide acetate cream is a topical antibiotic with good cartilage penetration; therefore, it can be used for the treatment of chondritis. Debridement of the involved, necrotic cartilage should be performed beforehand for adequate source control.[49]

BURN SEPSIS

Undiagnosed and untreated burn wound infection can lead to the conversion of partial-thickness wound to full thickness, and sepsis. High concentrations of bacteria in the burn wound, delayed presentation to a burn center, delayed removal of burned tissues, and decreased lean body mass increase the risk of sepsis. However, it should be

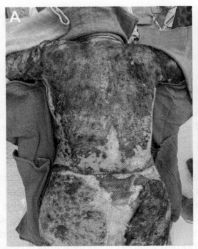
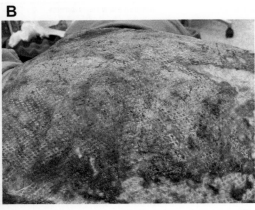

Fig. 2. (*A* and *B*) show the posterior trunk of a patient with 53% TBSA second-degree and third-degree burns developed biopsy-proven aspergillosis infection. (*Courtesy of* Francesco M. Egro, MD, Pittsburgh, PA.)

kept in mind that the source of sepsis in burn patients can be several other sources such as ventilator-associated pneumonia, central line associated blood stream infections, and catheter-associated urinary tract infections.[19,49]

Sepsis in burn patients is unique because it overlaps with the hypermetabolic response and systemic inflammatory response syndrome seen in all burn patients. Elevated temperature and tachycardia are a part of hypermetabolic response seen after burn injury as well as infection and sepsis. Furthermore, local changes such as erythema could be secondary to infection or burn itself. Therefore, the traditional criteria established for the diagnosis of sepsis might not be useful in burn patients.[49] In response, ABA defined specific criteria to diagnose sepsis in patients with burns[50] (**Table 2**). Once the patients meet at least 3 of these criteria, early, aggressive treatment with broad-spectrum antibiotics should be

initiated.[16,19] However, resistance to the commonly used antibiotics and prevalence of MDR organisms in burn units continues to be a challenge.[51] Therefore, the prevention of infections is the ultimate strategy to decrease the infection-related mortality in burn patients.[16,19]

PREVENTION OF BURN WOUND INFECTION

Prevention of burn wound infection is paramount because treatment of an established infection might be unsuccessful due to MDR and immunocompromised status of burn patients.[52,53] Initial prevention strategies include patient screening questionnaires before admission to the burn unit and full infection precautions on admission to minimize cross-contamination. The adoption of early excision and grafting of the burn wounds also reduced wound infection and improved burn outcomes.[9] Periodic surveillance swabs for MDR may help early diagnosis and treatment of infections in nonseptic patients.[16,53] Restoration of immune competence as early as possible is the mainstay of infection prevention in burn patients. Early enteral nutrition, early and complete excision of necrotic tissue and wound coverage, restrictive use of blood transfusion, early weaning from mechanical ventilation, antibiotic stewardship and restrictive use of invasive catheterization are all standard of care to restore immunologic barriers (**Box 2**).[38] Many modern burn centers have positive pressure isolation rooms as mentioned earlier in this article.[54,55] Isolating high-risk patients limits the spread of infections.[55] Strict hand hygiene, personal protective equipment, and limiting

---

> **Box 1**
> **Patient-specific risk factors for fungal infections**
>
> Increasing age
>
> Greater than 40% burned TBSA
>
> Inhalation injury
>
> Neutropenia
>
> Uncontrolled diabetes mellitus
>
> *Adapted from* Struck MF, Gille J. Fungal infections in burns: a comprehensive review. Ann Burns Fire Disasters. 2013;26(3):147-153.

Table 2
American Burn Association Consensus Definition of sepsis in burn patients

Temperature >39 or <36.5°C	
Progressive tachycardia	Adults >110 bpm, Children >2 SD above age-specific norms
Progressive tachypnea	Adults >25 bpm not ventilated, or minute ventilation >12 L/min ventilated. Children >2 SD above age-specific norms
Thrombocytopenia (will not apply until 3 d after initial resuscitation)	Adults <100,000/mcL. Children <2 SD below age-specific norms
Hyperglycemia (in the absence of preexisting diabetes mellitus)	Untreated plasma glucose >200 mg/dL or equivalent mM/L. Insulin resistance (eg, > 7 units of insulin per hour intravenous drip (adults), >25% increase in insulin requirements during 24 h)
Inability to continue enteral feedings >24 h	Abdominal distension, Enteral feeding intolerance (residual >150 mL/h in children or 2 times feeding rate in adults). Uncontrollable diarrhea (>2500 mL/d for adults or >400 mL/d for children)
Additional criteria: Positive cultures or pathologic examination tissue source, or clinical response to antimicrobials	

Abbreviations: bpm, beats per minute; SD, standard deviation.

Adapted from Greenhalgh DG, Saffle JR, Holmes JH 4th, Gamelli RL, Palmieri TL, Horton JW, Tompkins RG, Traber DL, Mozingo DW, Deitch EA, Goodwin CW, Herndon DN, Gallagher JJ, Sanford AP, Jeng JC, Ahrenholz DH, Neely AN, O'Mara MS, Wolf SE, Purdue GF, Garner WL, Yowler CJ, Latenser BA; American Burn Association Consensus Conference on Burn Sepsis and Infection Group. American Burn Association consensus conference to define sepsis and infection in burns. J Burn Care Res. 2007 Nov-Dec;28(6):776-90.

visitors are further precautionary measures to limit the spread of infections in burn units.

There is currently no evidence to support antimycotic or antibacterial prophylaxis for burn patients,[40,56,57] and an empiric use of broad-spectrum agents is not recommended due to the risk of generating MDR strains, increasing costs, as well as hepatotoxicity and nephrotoxicity.[48,58,59]

Topical Agents for Burn Wound Infection Prevention and Treatment

Several topical agents have emerged over the years to prevent or treat burn wound infections, and over the years, studies have demonstrated a reduction in morbidity and mortality.[60–62] Selection of the appropriate agent is based on the wound bed characteristics, antimicrobial spectrum, patient-related factors such as allergies or other contraindications, wound healing compromise, skin graft toxicity, and systemic toxicity. A list of topical agents can be found in **Table 3**.[63]

Avascular eschar covering burn wounds limits the delivery and accumulation of systemic antimicrobial agents at the wound.[59] Topical agents circumvent this problem by directly delivering

antimicrobial agents to the burn wound. Silver-based dressings are commonly used for infection prophylaxis in burn patients, and their antimicrobial properties is primarily due to their ability to release silver ions in the presence of moisture, which then interact with the microorganisms.[64–66]

Box 2
Best practices to decrease burn wound infections

Isolation

Hand hygiene and personal protective equipment

Decontamination of common areas for potential cross-contamination

Routine surveillance of hydrotherapy units, faucets, and other water sources

Early excision and grafting

Antibiotic stewardship[a]

Early enteral nutrition

[a]Avoid using broad-spectrum antibiotics before debridement because penetration will be poor.

Table 3
Topical antimicrobial agents used in burn treatment

Class	Agents	Antimicrobial Spectrum
Soaps	Johnson's baby shampoo	Broad-spectrum + biofilm
Oxidative halides	Dakin's solution (0.5%)	Broad-spectrum + biofilm
	Buffered Dakin's solution (0.025%)	Broad-spectrum + biofilm
	Oxychlorosene	Broad-spectrum + biofilm
	Hypochlorous acid	Broad-spectrum + biofilm
	Povidone-iodine	Broad-spectrum
Acids	Acetic acid (0.5%)	Bacteriostatic
	Acetic acid (2%)	Bacteriostatic
	Acetic acid (3%)	Bacteriostatic
Heavy metals	Silver nitrate 0.5%	Broad-spectrum
	Silver sulfadiazine (Silvadene)	Broad-spectrum
	Silver-releasing dressings	Broad-spectrum
	Xeroform-Bismuth tribromophenate	Limited bacteriostatic
	BIPPS-Bismuth subnitrate iodoform	Broad-spectrum
Antibiotics	Mafenide acetate (Sulfamylon)	Broad-spectrum
	Gentamycin sulfate (Gentamicin)	Broad-spectrum
	Bacitracin/polymyxin (Polysporin)	Broad-spectrum
	Nitrofurazone (Furacin)	Broad-spectrum[a]
	Mupirocin (Bactroban)	Broad-spectrum[a]
	Nystatin 100,000 U/g (Mycostatin)	Weak antifungal
	Nystatin 6,000,000 U/g	Strong antifungal

[a] No *Pseudomonas*.
Abbreviations: BIPPS, bismuth iodoform paraffin paste
Adapted from Dai T, Huang YY, Sharma SK, et al. Topical antimicrobials for burn wound infections. Recent Pat Antiinfect Drug Discov. 2010;5(2):124–151.

The main mechanisms of action include disruption of microorganisms' cell membranes, inhibition of microorganism's cellular enzymes involved in cellular respiration and other metabolic processes, microorganisms DNA damage limiting their ability to replicate and survive, and generation of reactive oxygen species causing oxidative stress and damage to various cellular components. Silver compounds come as solutions, creams, or bound to dressing materials. The most common of these agents is 1% silver sulfadiazine (SSD), which is a combination of silver nitrate and the antibiotic sodium sulfadiazine.[64] SSD is effective against *P aeruginosa* and has some activity against *C albicans*.[66] However, SSD may lead to the formation of a pseudo-eschar, which acts as a niche for bacterial proliferation. It is also associated with poor wound healing because it is highly toxic to keratinocytes and fibroblasts, and it is contraindicated in patients who have sulfa allergies.[67,68]

Bacitracin/polymyxin (Polysporin) ointment both acts as a topical antimicrobial that prevents bacterial growth over the skin grafts and as a lubricant that prevents mechanical shear plus maintains a moist wound environment needed for epithelial growth. Both bacitracin and polymyxin act by cell wall lysis but the concentrations are not high enough to treat established wound infections. For an increased antimicrobial activity, it can be used in combination with other topical agents, such as silver nitrate or mafenide. Although it is nontoxic, prolonged use may cause hypersensitivity reactions.[69]

Mupirocin (Bactroban, GSK, Australia, pseudomonic acid A) is derived from the *Pseudomonas fluorescens* capsule and acts via inhibition of bacterial protein synthesis. It is the topical treatment of choice for MRSA infections, gram-positive microbes, and intranasal MRSA decontamination. Mupirocin delays wound healing but significantly improves the final breaking strength of the wound. Recommended duration of treatment is less than 10 days due to rapid development of resistance.[60,69]

Mafenide acetate, also known as Sulfamylon, is an acetate salt form of mafenide, and it is available as cream or solution. The main mechanism of action includes bacterial growth inhibition, biofilm penetration, pH-dependent antimicrobial activity enhanced by an acidic environment. Mafenide acetate has the ability to penetrate biofilms, which enhances its efficacy in eradicating bacteria and preventing the formation of persistent infections in burn wounds. It is particularly good at penetrating eschars and, for this reason, is often used as a solution in full-thickness burns and as a topical cream for deep ear burns because of its efficacy in preventing chondritis. Although the cream can be used twice per day, the solution should be used to saturate gauze every 8 hours to remain above minimum inhibitory concentration (MIC). Mafenide acetate is a broad-spectrum antibiotic particularly effective against aerobic gram-negative bacilli, *P aeruginosa*, and anaerobes such as *Clostridium* species.[62,69] However, it has minimal activity against gram-positive aerobic bacteria such as *S aureus*.[60,62] Mafenide acetate can be painful, may cause metabolic acidosis due to is inhibitory effect of carbonic anhydrase, and is contraindicated in patients with sulfa allergies.

Gentamicin sulfate as 0.1% topical cream was introduced as a burn dressing, intended for antipseudomonal coverage of invasive burn wounds. Despite the theoretic advantages, the drug is readily absorbed through the burn wound and can reach to systemic levels to cause ototoxicity and nephrotoxicity. With the introduction of silver-containing ointments, routine use of gentamicin in burn patients has fallen out of favor. It should be reserved for patients whose wounds have become colonized with *P aeruginosa* because it may take as short as 3 weeks for *P aeruginosa* to develop resistance to gentamicin. Topical gentamicin might be an alternative to sulfa drugs in case of allergy to the latter.[70]

Vancomycin is a glycopeptide antibiotic that acts by inhibiting the cell wall biosynthesis of bacteria. It is considered as the first-line treatment of MRSA infections. It can be administered by intravenous and topical routes for the treatment of burn infections. Topical vancomycin is preferred over systemic formulations in case of a local wound infection to avoid the systemic side effects. Moreover, systemic vancomycin is less effective in the reduction of bacterial load in the wounds.[71,72] Several carrier molecules have been developed for the topical delivery of vancomycin to avoid the systemic side effects.[73,74]

A common drawback of antibiotic-based topical antimicrobial agents is the increased risk of fungal colonization with prolonged use. To minimize this risk, acetic acid (0.5%–5%) or sodium hypochlorite (0.0125%–0.5%) solution can be used. Acetic acid, also known as ethanoic acid, is a weak acid used as a disinfectant for skin and soft tissue infections. It has broad-spectrum antimicrobial activity and is especially effective against gram-negative bacteria (especially *P aeruginosa*). The main mechanism of action includes the disruption of microorganisms' cell membranes, inhibition of bacterial biofilm formation and growth, and pH-dependent antimicrobial activity enhanced by an acidic environment.[75]

Sodium hypochlorite is a chemical compound commonly used as bleach or household chlorine bleach. The diluted form (0.5%) is known as Dakin's solution and different strengths have been used in wound care. The main mechanism of action includes oxidative damage of cellular components, destruction of microorganisms' DNA and RNA limiting their ability to replicate and survive, and microorganism's cell membranes disruption. Sodium hypochlorite has broad-spectrum activity: Sodium hypochlorite is bactericidal against *S aureus*, methicillin-resistant staphylococci, enterococci, vancomycin-resistant enterococcus, *P aeruginosa*, and other gram-negative and gram-positive organisms; however, especially in high concentrations, sodium hypochlorite may be cytotoxic and be detrimental to wound healing.[62,69]

Topical antifungal agents may help treat local colonization and infection with fungi but they can also hide symptoms of ongoing infections.[33,76]

SYSTEMIC TREATMENT OF BURN INFECTIONS

Systemic broad-spectrum antimicrobials should be reserved for patients with cellulitis, invasive burn wound infections and sepsis. It is paramount, however, that any wound that is grossly infected or has an invasive infection is aggressively debrided to ensure all infected and necrotic tissue is excised. The antibiotic coverage should be narrowed as early as possible based on wound cultures, and the initial empiric antibiotic therapy should be based on facility-specific antibiogram and microbial resistance patterns as well as patient's length of stay.[55] The author's practice is to send biopsies and cultures to microbiology and pathology in wounds that are not suitable for autografting by postburn day 14, and on a weekly basis, until autografting is performed to ensure an early identification of invasive infection. Burn wound biopsy is also performed if there is significant drainage or discoloration of the wound, or when graft loss occurs unexpectedly.

Gram-positive organisms are the first to colonize burn wounds; therefore, septic patients early in the hospital stay are typically treated with penicillin, aminopenicillins, or penicillinase-resistant antibiotics such as methicillin, which have activity against gram-positive staphylococci and streptococci. However, early gram-negative infections are best treated with fourth-generation cephalosporins (eg, cefepime), carbapenems, or β-lactam–β-lactamase combination (eg, piperacillin tazobactam).[77,78] Later in the course of hospitalization gram-negative bacteria become dominant in burn wounds. Extended-spectrum penicillin and β-lactamase inhibitors or carbapenem can be used for the treatment of gram-negative infections with the addition of vancomycin if MRSA is suspected. Aminoglycosides should be added for MDR *P aeruginosa* infections. If vancomycin-resistant organisms such as VRE are common in the microbiome of the facility, linezolid or a combination of ampicillin and an aminoglycoside is the antibiotic option.[77,78]

The risk of MDR infection is directly correlated with burn severity, length of hospital stay, and prolonged use of systemic antibiotics.[79–81] The incidence of MDR infections may increase more than 5 times only after 4 weeks of hospitalization compared with first week of hospitalization.[78–83] The pillars of treatment of confirmed MDR bacterial infections are source control and initiation of appropriate broad-spectrum antibiotics as soon as possible.[15] The International Society for Burn Injury practice guidelines advise a facility-specific antibiotic stewardship program to guide the antibiotic treatment.[84,85] Antibiotic dosing should consider the hyperdynamic state in burn patients, which increases renal clearance of commonly administered antibiotics.[80,81]

Invasive fungal infections (eg, aspergillosis and zygomycosis) are a major challenge for burn surgeons. These infections can be mistaken for early bacterial burn wound infection, and a delay of identifying the causative fungus species may delay appropriate treatment. An increasing number of uncommon and resistant fungal pathogens have been reported. Early aggressive excision and wound closure play crucial role, especially in preventing infections caused by yeasts and molds or any other agent. This needs to be combined with topical and systemic therapy because they have high mortality rates.[85–89] In the case of invasive *Aspergillus* infection, the use of voriconazole is the first-choice therapy, whereas *Mucor* infection is typically treated with amphotericin. *Candida* species are treated with triazoles (eg, fluconazole and voriconazole) and echinocandins (eg, caspofungin). The author's preference to treat invasive fungal infections involves aggressive surgical debridement combined with topical antifungal and antibacterial solutions (amphotericin B, vancomycin, and gentamicin), and intravenous antifungal therapy based on sensitivity.[89]

SUMMARY

Infection remains the greatest source of morbidity following burn injury. Aggressive preventive measures and prompt treatment are essential to mitigate this life-threatening complication. Eschar and necrotic tissue are a nidus for pathogens proliferation. Burns need to be promptly excised and autografted to improve healing outcomes and minimize infection proliferation. The longer reepithelialization is delayed, the greater the susceptibility to infection and the potential for colonization of resistant organisms. Various strategies have proven to minimize colonization between burn injury and autografting. Source control can be achieved through meticulous washing and debridement of the affected area in hydrotherapy, application of topical antimicrobial agents, and close clinical and microbiological monitoring of burn tissue. Sepsis and septic shock need to be diagnosed and treated promptly with broad-spectrum antibiotics followed by targeted therapy once sensitivities are back. Invasive fungal infection remains a great challenge for burn surgeons due to its high morbidity and mortality rate. Early diagnosis is key, and aggressive measures have to be adopted to optimize outcomes. Future directions in the management of burn wound infections include the development of new topical antimicrobial agents and antifungal drugs to battle against resistant pathogens and fungal infections. To ensure effective management of burn wounds, it is important to establish consistent and standardized testing methods in clinical microbiology laboratories. These methods would enable routine testing of bacterial isolates from burn wounds for susceptibility to the topical antimicrobial agents available at a specific burn center. Additionally, implementing a rotation program for the use of topical antimicrobial agents may help reduce the development of resistance. The fight against burn wound infection will only be victorious due to the collaborative efforts between infectious disease specialists, clinical microbiology laboratories, burn centers, and health-care professionals.

CLINICS CARE POINTS

- Be alert about the signs and symptoms of sepsis in burn patients because the clinical picture may not fit the classic definition of sepsis.
- Make sure patients are resuscitated adequately before any surgical procedure.
- In case of an outbreak, check the shared areas and surfaces first to determine the source of infection.
- Try to avoid interruption in the nutrition of the patients.

DISCLOSURE

The authors have no disclosures.

REFERENCES

1. Barrow RE, Spies M, Barrow LN, et al. Influence of demographics and inhalation injury on burn mortality in children. Burns 2004;30(1):72–7.
2. National Burn Repository Chicago 2016 Available at: https://ameriburn.org/wpcontent/uploads/2017/05/2016abanbr_final_42816.pdf. Accessed June 30, 2023.
3. Kargozar S, Mozafari M, Hamzehlou S, et al. Using Bioactive Glasses in the management of burns. Front Bioeng Biotechnol 2019;7:62.
4. Corcione S, Pensa A, Castiglione A, et al. Epidemiology, prevalence and risk factors for infections in burn patients: results from a regional burn centre's analysis. J Chemother 2021;33(1):62–6.
5. Mir MA, Khurram MF, Khan AH. What should be the antibiotic prescription protocol for burn patients admitted in the department of burns, plastic and reconstructive surgery. Int Wound J 2017;14(1):194–7.
6. Maslova E, Eisaiankhongi L, Sjöberg F, et al. Burns and biofilms: priority pathogens and in vivo models. NPJ Biofilms Microbiomes 2021;7(1):73.
7. Hidalgo F, Mas D, Rubio M, et al. Infections in critically ill burn patients. Med Intensiva 2016;40(3):179–85.
8. Tiwari VK. Burn wound: How it differs from other wounds? Indian J Plast Surg 2012;45(2):364–73.
9. Wang Y, Beekman J, Hew J, et al. Burn injury: Challenges and advances in burn wound healing, infection, pain and scarring. Adv Drug Deliv Rev 2018;123:3–17.
10. Gonzalez MR, Ducret V, Leoni S, et al. Transcriptome analysis of *Pseudomonas aeruginosa* cultured in Human burn wound exudates. Front Cell Infect Microbiol 2018;8:39.
11. Neely AN, Fowler LA, Kagan RJ, et al. Procalcitonin in pediatric burn patients: an early indicator of sepsis? J Burn Care Rehabil 2004;25(1):76–80.
12. Erol S, Altoparlak U, Akcay MN, et al. Changes of microbial flora and wound colonization in burned patients. Burns 2004;30(4):357–61.
13. Manson WL, Klasen HJ, Sauer EW, et al. Selective intestinal decontamination for prevention of wound colonization in severely burned patients: a retrospective analysis. Burns 1992;18(2):98–102.
14. Nasser S, Mabrouk A, Maher A. Colonization of burn wounds in Ain Shams University burn Unit. Burns 2003;29(3):229–33.
15. Church D, Elsayed S, Reid O, et al. Burn wound infections. Clin Microbiol Rev 2006;19(2):403–34.
16. Vinaik R, Barayan D, Shahrokhi S, et al. Management and prevention of drug resistant infections in burn patients. Expert Rev Anti Infect Ther 2019;17(8):607–19.
17. Baj J, Korona-Głowniak I, Buszewicz G, et al. Viral infections in burn patients: a state-of-the-Art review. Viruses 2020;12(11):1315.
18. Singer M, Deutschman CS, Seymour CW, et al. The third International consensus definitions for sepsis and septic shock (Sepsis-3). JAMA 2016;315(8):801–10.
19. Greenhalgh DG. Sepsis in the burn patient: a different problem than sepsis in the general population. Burns Trauma 2017;5:23.
20. Powers JH. Development of drugs for antimicrobial-resistant pathogens. Curr Opin Infect Dis 2003;16(6):547–51.
21. Williams FN, Lee JO. Pediatric burn infection. Surg Infect 2021;22(1):54–7.
22. Ramakrishnan M, Putli Bai S, Babu M. Study on biofilm formation in burn wound infection in a pediatric hospital in Chennai, India. Ann Burns Fire Disasters 2016;29(4):276–80.
23. Taneja N, Chari P, Singh M, et al. Evolution of bacterial flora in burn wounds: key role of environmental disinfection in control of infection. Int J Burns Trauma 2013;3(2):102–7.
24. Percival SL, McCarty SM, Lipsky B. Biofilms and wounds: an Overview of the evidence. Adv Wound Care 2015;4(7):373–81.
25. Flemming HC, Wingender J, Szewzyk U, et al. Biofilms: an emergent form of bacterial life. Nat Rev Microbiol 2016;14(9):563–75.
26. Rumbaugh KP, Sauer K. Biofilm dispersion. Nat Rev Microbiol 2020;18(10):571–86.
27. Mah TF, O'Toole GA. Mechanisms of biofilm resistance to antimicrobial agents. Trends Microbiol 2001;9(1):34–9.
28. Bjarnsholt T, Kirketerp-Møller K, Jensen PØ, et al. Why chronic wounds will not heal: a novel hypothesis. Wound Repair Regen 2008;16(1):2–10.
29. Moser C, Jensen PØ, Thomsen K, et al. Immune responses to *Pseudomonas aeruginosa* biofilm infections. Front Immunol 2021;12:625597.
30. Garcia Garcia JA, Gonzalez Chavez AM, Orozco Grados JJ. Topical antimicrobial agents for the prevention of burn-wound infection. What Do International guidelines Recommend? A systematic review. World J Plast Surg 2022;11(3):3–12.
31. Lachiewicz AM, Hauck CG, Weber DJ, et al. Bacterial infections after burn injuries: Impact of multidrug resistance. Clin Infect Dis 2017;65(12):2130–6.
32. Carr JA, Phillips BD, Bowling WM. The utility of bronchoscopy after inhalation injury complicated by pneumonia in burn patients: results from the National Burn Repository. J Burn Care Res 2009;30(6):967–74.
33. Branski LK, Al-Mousawi A, Rivero H, et al. Emerging infections in burns. Surg Infect 2009;10(5):389–97.
34. Robson MC, Krizek TJ. Predicting skin graft survival. J Trauma 1973;13(3):213–7.

35. Guggenheim M, Zbinden R, Handschin AE, et al. Changes in bacterial isolates from burn wounds and their antibiograms: a 20-year study (1986-2005). Burns 2009;35(4):553–60.

36. Hodle AE, Richter KP, Thompson RM. Infection control practices in U.S. burn units. J Burn Care Res 2006;27(2):142–51.

37. Altoparlak U, Erol S, Akcay MN, et al. The time-related changes of antimicrobial resistance patterns and predominant bacterial profiles of burn wounds and body flora of burned patients. Burns 2004; 30(7):660–4.

38. Vonberg RP, Gastmeier P. Nosocomial aspergillosis in outbreak settings. J Hosp Infect 2006;63(3): 246–54.

39. Struck MF, Gille J. Fungal infections in burns: a comprehensive review. Ann Burns Fire Disasters 2013;26(3):147–53.

40. Jarvis WR. Epidemiology of nosocomial fungal infections, with emphasis on Candida species. Clin Infect Dis 1995;20(6):1526–30.

41. Ballard J, Edelman L, Saffle J, et al. Positive fungal cultures in burn patients: a multicenter review. J Burn Care Res 2008;29(1):213–21.

42. Mousa HA, Al-Bader SM, Hassan DA. Correlation between fungi isolated from burn wounds and burn care units. Burns 1999;25(2):145–7.

43. Kealey GP, Heinle JA, Lewis RW, et al. Value of the Candida antigen assay in diagnosis of systemic candidiasis in burn patients. J Trauma 1992;32(3):285–8.

44. Luo G, Peng Y, Yuan Z, et al. Yeast from burn patients at a major burn centre of China. Burns 2011; 37(2):299–303.

45. Gore DC, Chinkes D, Heggers J, et al. Association of hyperglycemia with increased mortality after severe burn injury. J Trauma 2001;51(3):540–4.

46. Trupkovic T, Gille J, Fischer H, et al. Antimikrobielle Therapie bei Patienten nach Verbrennungstrauma [Antimicrobial treatment in burn injury patients]. Anaesthesist 2012;61(3):249–58.

47. Ekenna O, Fader RC. Effect of thermal injury and immunosuppression on the dissemination of Candida albicans from the mouse gastrointestinal tract. J Burn Care Rehabil 1989;10(2):138–45.

48. Rodloff C, Koch D, Schaumann R. Epidemiology and antifungal resistance in invasive candidiasis. Eur J Med Res 2011;16(4):187–95.

49. Schofield CM, Murray CK, Horvath EE, et al. Correlation of culture with histopathology in fungal burn wound colonization and infection. Burns 2007; 33(3):341–6.

50. Greenhalgh DG, Saffle JR, Holmes JH 4th, et al. American burn association consensus conference on burn sepsis and infection Group. American burn association consensus conference to define sepsis and infection in burns. J Burn Care Res 2007;28(6): 776–90.

51. Ladhani HA, Yowler CJ, Claridge JA. Burn wound colonization, infection, and sepsis. Surg Infect 2021;22(1):44–8.

52. Norbury W, Herndon DN, Tanksley J, et al. Infection in burns. Surg Infect 2016;17(2):250–5.

53. Merchant N, Smith K, Jeschke MG. An Ounce of prevention Saves Tons of Lives: infection in burns. Surg Infect 2015;16(4):380–7.

54. Rutala WA, Weber DJ. Are room decontamination units needed to prevent transmission of environmental pathogens? Infect Control Hosp Epidemiol 2011;32(8):743–7.

55. Dansby W, Purdue G, Hunt J, et al. Aerosolization of methicillin-resistant Staphylococcus aureus during an epidemic in a burn intensive care unit. J Burn Care Res 2008;29(2):331–7.

56. Rosenberger LH, Hranjec T, Politano AD, et al. Effective cohorting and "superisolation" in a single intensive care unit in response to an outbreak of diverse multi-drug-resistant organisms. Surg Infect 2011; 12(5):345–50.

57. Moore EC, Padiglione AA, Wasiak J, et al. Candida in burns: risk factors and outcomes. J Burn Care Res 2010;31(2):257–63.

58. O'Driscoll T, Crank CW. Vancomycin-resistant enterococcal infections: epidemiology, clinical manifestations, and optimal management. Infect Drug Resist 2015;8:217–30.

59. Eggimann P, Lamoth F, Marchetti O. On track to limit antifungal overuse! Intensive Care Med 2009;35(4): 582–4 [published correction appears in Intensive Care Med. 2009 Apr;35(4):772].

60. Greenhalgh DG. Topical antimicrobial agents for burn wounds. Clin Plast Surg 2009;36(4):597–606.

61. Glasser JS, Guymon CH, Mende K, et al. Activity of topical antimicrobial agents against multidrug-resistant bacteria recovered from burn patients. Burns 2010;36(8):1172–84.

62. Dai T, Huang YY, Sharma SK, et al. Topical antimicrobials for burn wound infections. Recent Pat Anti-Infect Drug Discov 2010;5(2):124–51.

63. Cambiaso-Daniel J, Gallagher JJ, Norbury WB, et al. Chapter 11 - treatment of infection in burns. In: Herndon DN, editor. Total burn care. 4th edition. Amsterdam, Netherlands: Elsevier; 2012. p. 93–113.e2.

64. Storm-Versloot MN, Vos CG, Ubbink DT, et al. Topical silver for preventing wound infection. Cochrane Database Syst Rev 2010;3:CD006478.

65. Marx DE, Barillo DJ. Silver in medicine: the basic science. Burns 2014;40(Suppl 1):S9–18.

66. Dunn K, Edwards-Jones V. The role of Acticoat with nanocrystalline silver in the management of burns. Burns 2004;30(Suppl 1):S1–9.

67. Wasiak J, Cleland H, Campbell F, et al. Dressings for superficial and partial thickness burns. Cochrane Database Syst Rev 2013;2013(3):CD002106.

68. Duc QI, Breetveld M, Middelkoop E, et al. A cytotoxic analysis of antiseptic medication on skin substitutes and autograft. Br J Dermatol 2007; 157(1):33–40.

69. Monafo WW, West MA. Current treatment recommendations for topical burn therapy. Drugs 1990; 40(3):364–73.

70. Snelling CF, Ronald AR, Waters WR, et al. Comparison of silver sulfadiazine and gentamicin for topical prophylaxis against burn wound sepsis. Can Med Assoc J 1978;119(5):466–70.

71. Vingsbo Lundberg C, Frimodt-Møller N. Efficacy of topical and systemic antibiotic treatment of meticillin-resistant Staphylococcus aureus in a murine superficial skin wound infection model. Int J Antimicrob Agents 2013;42(3):272–5.

72. Sevgi M, Toklu A, Vecchio D, et al. Topical antimicrobials for burn infections - an update. Recent Pat Anti-Infect Drug Discov 2013;8(3):161–97.

73. Kausar R, Khan AU, Jamil B, et al. Development and pharmacological evaluation of vancomycin loaded chitosan films. Carbohydr Polym 2021;256:117565.

74. Giandalia G, De Caro V, Cordone L, et al. Trehalose-hydroxyethylcellulose microspheres containing vancomycin for topical drug delivery. Eur J Pharm Biopharm 2001;52(1):83–9.

75. Halstead FD, Rauf M, Moiemen NS, et al. The antibacterial activity of acetic acid against biofilm-Producing pathogens of Relevance to burns patients. PLoS One 2015;10(9):e0136190.

76. Heggers JP, Robson MC, Herndon DN, et al. The efficacy of nystatin combined with topical microbial agents in the treatment of burn wound sepsis. J Burn Care Rehabil 1989;10(6):508–11.

77. Avni T, Levcovich A, Ad-El DD, et al. Prophylactic antibiotics for burns patients: systematic review and meta-analysis. BMJ 2010;340:c241.

78. van Duin D, Strassle PD, DiBiase LM, et al. Timeline of health care-associated infections and pathogens after burn injuries. Am J Infect Control 2016;44(12): 1511–6.

79. ISBI Practice Guidelines Committee; Steering Subcommittee; Advisory Subcommittee. ISBI practice guidelines for burn care. Burns 2016;42(5): 953–1021.

80. Silvestri L, van Saene HK, Milanese M, et al. Selective decontamination of the digestive tract reduces bacterial bloodstream infection and mortality in critically ill patients. Systematic review of randomized, controlled trials. J Hosp Infect 2007;65(3):187–203.

81. Girerd-Genessay I, Bénet T, Vanhems P. Multidrug-resistant bacterial outbreaks in burn Units: a Synthesis of the literature According to the ORION Statement. J Burn Care Res 2016;37(3):172–80.

82. Wanis M, Walker SAN, Daneman N, et al. Impact of hospital length of stay on the distribution of Gram negative bacteria and likelihood of isolating a resistant organism in a Canadian burn center. Burns 2016;42(1):104–11.

83. Kanamori H, Parobek CM, Juliano JJ, et al. A prolonged outbreak of KPC-3-Producing Enterobacter cloacae and Klebsiella pneumoniae Driven by multiple mechanisms of resistance transmission at a large Academic burn center. Antimicrob Agents Chemother 2017;61(2). e01516-16.

84. Barlam TF, Cosgrove SE, Abbo LM, et al. Implementing an antibiotic stewardship program: guidelines by the infectious diseases Society of America and the Society for healthcare epidemiology of America. Clin Infect Dis 2016;62(10):e51–77.

85. Wagner B, Filice GA, Drekonja D, et al. Antimicrobial stewardship programs in inpatient hospital settings: a systematic review. Infect Control Hosp Epidemiol 2014;35(10):1209–28.

86. Palackic A, Popp D, Tapking C, et al. Fungal infections in burn patients. Surg Infect 2021;22(1):83–7. https://doi.org/10.1089/sur.2020.299.

87. Murray CK, Loo FL, Hospenthal DR, et al. Incidence of systemic fungal infection and related mortality following severe burns. Burns 2008;34(8):1108–12.

88. Ledgard JP, van Hal S, Greenwood JE. Primary cutaneous zygomycosis in a burns patient: a review. J Burn Care Res 2008;29(2):286–90.

89. Greenhalgh DG. Management of burns. N Engl J Med 2019;380(24):2349–59.

Pain Management in Burn Patients

Pharmacologic Management of Acute and Chronic Pain

Kevin M. Klifto, DO, PharmD[a],*, C. Scott Hultman, MD, MBA[b]

KEYWORDS

- Analgesia • Burn • Neuropathic • Nociceptive • Nociplastic • Pain
- Peripheral nervous system diseases

KEY POINTS

- Burn-related pain should be assessed first by chronicity (acute or chronic), followed by type (nociceptive, neuropathic, nociplastic) to guide multimodal pharmacologic management in a stepwise algorithm approach.
- Multimodal pharmacologic management includes knowledge and understanding of pharmacokinetics, pharmacodynamics, pharmacoeconomics, pharmacogenomics, and pharmacotherapeutics.
- Combination therapy increases efficacy and reduces toxicity by offering a multimodal approach to burn-related pain by targeting different receptors in the peripheral nervous system (PNS) and central nervous system (CNS).
- Responses to multimodal pharmacologic management should frequently be assessed using the numerical rating scale (NRS) for pain (mild = 1–3; moderate = 4–6; severe = 7–10).
- Consider etiologies of burn-related pain that may be amenable to surgical interventions or chronic pain states that may require a referral to pain management.

DEFINITION OF PAIN

Pain following a burn injury or burn-related pain can contribute to decreased quality of life (QOL) and long-term patient morbidity, limiting functional recovery. Pain was redefined in 2020 by the International Association for the Study of Pain Subcommittee as an unpleasant sensory and emotional experience associated with, or resembling that associated with, actual or potential tissue damage.[1] Pain is always a personal experience that is influenced to varying degrees by biological, psychological, and social factors.[1]

Sensory structures are contained within the skin dermis. They consist of free nerve endings (pain, temperature, and touch), Meissner's corpuscles (light discriminatory touch), and Pacinian corpuscles (pressure). Pain signals are transmitted by free nerve endings of the peripheral nervous system (PNS) through myelinated $A\delta$ fibers (fast pain) and unmyelinated C fibers (slow and chronic pain). Signals synapse in the central nervous system (CNS) at the dorsal horn of the spinal cord. Fibers cross midline within the spinal cord to ascend to the thalamus through the lateral spinothalamic tracts, followed by the post-central gyrus, where conscious perception of the stimulus may occur.[2] Pharmacologic agents target various receptor pathways within the CNS and PNS to reduce pain.

All burn injuries may result in burn-related pain. Pruritus or itching can be an unbearable component of burn-related pain. The prevalence of pruritus

[a] Division of Plastic and Reconstructive Surgery, Department of Surgery, University of Missouri Health Care, 1 Hospital Drive, Columbia, MO 65212, USA; [b] Department of Plastic and Reconstructive Surgery, WPP Plastic and Reconstructive Surgery, WakeMed Health and Hospitals, 3000 New Bern Avenue, Raleigh, NC 27610, USA
* Corresponding author. Division of Plastic and Reconstructive Surgery, Department of Surgery, University of Missouri Health Care, 1 Hospital Drive, Columbia, MO 65212, USA.
E-mail address: author.kklifto@gmail.com

Clin Plastic Surg 51 (2024) 267–301
https://doi.org/10.1016/j.cps.2023.11.004

following a burn has been reported ranging from 67% to 87%.[3] Burn-related pain results from stimulation of skin nociceptors that respond to thermal, mechanical, and chemical stimuli. Stimuli are transmitted from the PNS to the CNS through afferent Aδ fibers and C fibers. Nerves that remain uninjured and exposed during first and second degree, or superficial/deep and partial-thickness burns will generate pain throughout the time of recovery. Nerve endings destroyed in the dermis of third degree or full-thickness burns will not transmit immediate pain signals. Patients may still initially complain of unlocalized deep or dull pain and later localized sharp pain.

ASSESSMENT OF PAIN

Rating scales are used to objectively quantify, assess, measure, and monitor the subjective nature of pain. In addition, rating scales measure changes in pain scores to help determine responses and direct interventions. Validated scales include the Visual Analogue Scale (VAS), the Numerical Rating Scale (NRS), the Verbal Rating Scale (VRS), and the Faces Pain Scale-Revised.[4] Numerous studies demonstrate that the NRS is preferred due to ease of use, higher compliance rates, better responsiveness and good applicability compared to the VAS and VRS.[5] Clinicians should ensure patients understand how to interpret the pain severity scale. Pain scores 1 to 3 are considered mild, 4 to 6 are considered moderate, and 7 to 10 are considered severe pain (Fig. 1). As pain severity increases and becomes moderate to severe, stronger pharmacologic agents such as opioids may be appropriate management for short durations. Frequent assessments should be made to determine responses to management, along with the characteristics and severity of burn-related pain. Consider etiologies of burn-related pain that may be amenable to surgical interventions to avoid unnecessary chronic systemic drug exposure.[6]

ACUTE AND CHRONIC PAIN

The chronicity of burn-related pain should first be assessed. Burn-related pain may be classified as acute or chronic, defined by the duration of pain. Pain becomes chronic if left untreated or when no etiologies are identified to treat.

- *Acute pain* is defined as self-limiting or pain $\leq$ 6 months duration.
- *Chronic pain* is defined as pain > 6 months duration.

In the acute phases of pain following burn injury, burn management, or even at discharge from the

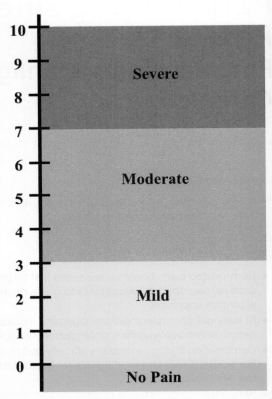

Fig. 1. Numerical Rating Scale (NRS) for Burn-related Pain. Pain is categorized as mild, moderate, and severe (mild = 1–3; moderate = 4–6; severe = 7–10).

burn unit, it may be difficult to differentiate burn-related acute nociceptive pain from neuropathic pain. Overlap between burn-related nociceptive and neuropathic pain is common during the acute setting. While in the chronic phases of pain following burn injury, it may be difficult to differentiate burn-related chronic neuropathic pain from nociplastic pain.

TYPES OF PAIN

Once the chronicity has been assessed and established as burn-related acute or chronic pain, the type should be assessed and established. Choosing appropriate burn-related multimodal pharmacologic targeted pain management requires that the pain being treated is correctly diagnosed and classified as nociceptive, neuropathic, and/or nociplastic pain.[1]

- *Nociceptive pain* is defined as pain secondary to peripheral sources of noxious stimulation or inflammatory mediators, processed by a normal somatosensory system.
- *Neuropathic pain* is defined as pain secondary to a lesion or disease process involving the CNS or PNS, resulting in an abnormal somatosensory system.

- *Nociplastic pain* is defined as pain characterized by clinical and psychophysical findings that suggest altered nociception, despite there being no clear evidence of actual or threatened tissue damage causing the activation of nociceptors or evidence for disease or lesion of the somatosensory system causing chronic pain.

Acute Nociceptive Pain

The most severe nociceptive pain for a burned patient often occurs during dressing changes and the first several days following surgery. Nociceptive pain can result in musculoskeletal pain. Analgesics and anesthetics should be administered prior to performing dressing changes. Staff should always minimize pain by avoiding unnecessary stimuli.

Nociceptive pruritus is mediated through free nerve endings of the PNS that sense environmental stimuli within the skin. Non-neuron cells of the surrounding tissues in the skin secrete itch-inducing substances that activate primary afferent C-fibers.[7] Sensations of pruritus are transmitted by substance P and calcitonin gene-related peptide through pruritus-selective, unmyelinated, histamine-sensitive, C nerve fibers with a small diameter and a slow delivery rate.[3] Secondary neurons ascend to the ventromedial and dorsomedial nuclei of the thalamus, resulting in the desire to scratch an itch.[7]

Acute or Chronic Neuropathic Pain

Burn-related acute or chronic neuropathic pain is a manifestation related either to the burn injury itself or to management of the burn injury resulting in direct injury or irritation to a nerve with subsequent signs and symptoms of pain.[6,8–11] Burn-related neuropathic pain may be classified by its etiology to guide patient management, with the goal of improving pain outcomes. Etiologies of neuropathic pain consist of direct nerve injury, nerve compression, electrical injury, and nerve dysfunction secondary to systemic injury.[6]

Neuropathic pruritus may be mediated through injury to the PNS or CNS. Peripheral afferent nerves become sensitized and result in altered input to the CNS.[7] Sensitized nociceptors develop spontaneous activity when injured, resulting in molecular changes and the release of chemical substances. C-fibers have the largest innervation territories.[12] Proximal inflammation within injured nerves and nerve roots contribute to boundary enlargement of C-fibers boundaries, allowing the sensation of pruritus beyond the innervation areas of injured nerves.[12] Nerve injury can increase the activity of dorsal horn projection neurons, decrease afferent inhibition, and decrease CNS

inhibitory neurons which include gamma-aminobutyric acid (GABA) interneurons.[7]

Approximately 8% of the burn population will likely develop burn-related acute neuropathic pain at 3 months,[10] while 6% of the burn population will likely progress to chronic neuropathic pain, persisting beyond 6 months.[9] Predictors of burn-related chronic neuropathic pain differ by anatomic locations of burns.[8] A patient's risk of developing burn-related chronic neuropathic pain at 6 months may accurately be calculated using a validated predictive model.[8] The strongest predictors are age, tobacco use, substance abuse, alcohol abuse, upper arm burns, thigh burns, number of burn-related operations, and hospital length of stay.[8]

Chronic Nociplastic Pain

A burns potent inflammatory response can result in nociplastic primary hyperalgesia at the level of the PNS by releasing inflammatory mediators that sensitize active nociceptors at the area of burn injury. If the epidermis is removed or destroyed, nerve endings may be exposed and susceptible to stimulation. Repeated stimulation of nociceptive afferent fibers can result in nociplastic secondary hyperalgesia at the level of the CNS by increasing the sensitivity in uninjured tissues mediated through the spinal cord. Injured nerves will generate neuropathic pain throughout the time of recovery.

Burn-related chronic nociplastic pain results in pathophysiologic primary and/or secondary sensitization and subsequent neuromodulation that requires management through mechanisms of relearning. Elevated concentrations of endogenous opioids can worsen hyperalgesia and alter sleep architecture, leading to opioid-induced hyperalgesia (OIH).[13,14] The development and maintenance of pain hypersensitivity has also been found to be dependent on activation of the N-methyl-D-aspartate (NMDA) receptor.[15] Indirectly and directly targeting the NMDA receptor has proven effective for managing nociplastic pain.[16–19]

Nociplastic pruritus develops from environmental stimuli within the skin and continues to stimulate nociceptors. Environmental stimuli may result from cellular responses and inflammatory mediators as the body attempts to heal. Hypertrophic and hyperproliferative scars can continue to release mediators through cells involved in tissue remodeling. Mediators stimulate the PNS, followed by the CNS, resulting in sensitization, and altered nociception.[7]

BURN-RELATED PATHOPHYSIOLOGIC PHASES

Burn-related pathophysiologic phases will alter drug pharmacokinetics and pharmacodynamics. Percent total body surface area (%TBSA) burns more than 20% in adults (>15% in pediatrics and geriatrics), result in both local effects at and around the site of burn injury and systemic effects involving uninjured tissues. Systemic effects occur in 2 acute sequential phases that may potentially alter the pharmacokinetics and pharmacodynamics of drugs.[20]

Phase 1 (Shock Phase)

Phase 1, or the shock (ebb) phase occurs over the first 48 hours.[20] Burned tissues release inflammatory mediators that cause local vasodilatation, vascular hyperpermeability and extracellular matrix destruction. Tissues become more permeable to proteins, which alter fluid gradients. Fluids shift from the blood vessels into the surrounding tissue, resulting in severe hypovolemia. Cardiac output decreases, systemic vascular resistance increases and blood flow to all organs decreases. Poor blood flow to the kidneys decreases the glomerular filtration rate (GFR) and urine output. During the first phase, pharmacokinetics is altered by decreasing drug distribution rates and decreasing the creatinine clearance (CrCl).[21]

Phase 2 (Hypermetabolic Phase)

Phase 2, or the hypermetabolic (flow) phase, follows from the systemic effects of inflammation and oxidative stress.[20] Cardiac output increases, systemic vascular resistance decreases, and blood flow to all organs increases. Blood flow to the kidneys increases, causing an increased GFR and CrCl. Blood flow also increases to the liver; however, due to ongoing hepatic dysfunction, metabolism by cytochrome P450 (CYP450), oxidation, reduction, and hydroxylation reactions are decreased. Plasma protein binding of drugs is altered by reduced carrier protein synthesis, resulting in higher concentrations of unbound drug. Changes in physiologic parameters will result in pharmacokinetic alterations.[21]

PHARMACOKINETICS

Drug absorption, distribution, metabolism, and excretion may all change following burn injury.[22] Phase 1 and phase 2 pathophysiologic changes are important considerations for burn-related pain. They will alter normal drug pharmacokinetics and pharmacodynamics (**Table 1**).[21]

Absorption

Absorption changes during phase 1 with increased intestinal permeability and decreased blood flow to the gastrointestinal tract. Decreased blood flow delays absorption, resulting in decreased peak drug concentrations and decreased drug bioavailability. Gastric pH decreases, acidity increases, and alterations in drug dissociation or dissolution may be seen. During phase 2, intestinal permeability remains increased, while blood flow to the gastrointestinal tract now increases, resulting in increased absorption of oral drugs and increased systemic concentrations.[21,22]

Distribution

Distribution changes with membrane permeability, shifts in intracellular and extracellular volumes and drug binding proteins. As membrane permeability increases, highly protein bound drugs that normally remain in the plasma with low volumes of distributions, may achieve higher volumes of distribution and accumulate in tissues. For drugs that are normally highly protein bound with small volumes of distribution, loading doses may need to be administered to compensate for altered pharmacokinetics to achieve similar plasma drug concentrations. Decreased plasma concentrations of albumin can increase the unbound fraction of acidic and neutral pH drugs, while decreased plasma concentrations of α1-acidglycoprotein can increase the unbound fraction of basic pH drugs. This can further alter a drugs volume of distribution. Major changes in pharmacokinetics can be seen with drugs that are highly protein bound, have a narrow therapeutic index, or minimal first-pass metabolism.[21,22]

Metabolism

Metabolism is decreased, even during the hypermetabolic burn state secondary to hepatic dysfunction. Peak hepatic dysfunction occurs 5 to 10 days following the initial burn injury. Phase I CYP450 liver metabolism (oxidation, reduction, and hydroxylation) is decreased, while phase II liver metabolism (conjugation) remains unaffected.[21] Drugs that normally undergo high first-pass phase I metabolism may enter the systemic circulation at toxic concentrations, while drugs that undergo phase II metabolism may have subtherapeutic concentrations secondary to increased blood flow to the liver. Activities of the plasma enzymes acetylcholinesterase and pseudo-cholinesterase are decreased. Drugs may have prolonged circulation resulting in longer elimination half-lives. Pharmacogenomics are important for identifying different metabolic gene expressions that may alter an individual's clinical response to a drug.[23]

Excretion

Excretion is decreased during the first 48 hours with decreased renal blood flow, GFR, and CrCl.[21] Once

Table 1
Normal adult drug pharmacokinetics for pain management

Drug	Absorption	Distribution	Metabolism	Excretion
Acetaminophen/ paracetamol	PO: small intestine (rate dependent on gastric emptying): stomach PR: delayed, erratic absorption Onset of action: PO:<1h; IV:5–10 min	Time to peak: PO: IR:10–60 min; IV:15 min Protein binding:10%–25%; Vd:0.8 ± 0.2 L/kg Peak effect: IV:1h Duration: PO, IV:4-6h	Hepatic: sulfate and glucuronide conjugates, CYP2E1 to toxic intermediate, NAPQI, conjugated rapidly with glutathione, inactivated to nontoxic cysteine and mercapturic acid conjugates; major CYP2E1 substrate	Urine:<5% unchanged, 60%–80% glucuronide metabolites, 20%–30% sulfate metabolites, 8% cysteine, mercapturic acid metabolites Half-life:2.4 ± 0.6 h; CrCl<30:2-5h
Ibuprofen	PO: rapid (85%) Bioavailability:80% Onset of action: PO:30–60 min	Time to peak: tablets:1-2h; suspension:1h Protein binding:>99%; Vd: PO:0.12 L/kg	Hepatic: oxidation; inactive R-isomer slowly and incompletely (60%) converted to active S-isomer; inhibits OAT1/3	Urine:45%–80% metabolites, 1% unchanged drug, 14% conjugated; feces Half-life: PO:2h; IV:2–2.5 h; R-enantiomer:10h; S-enantiomer:25h ESRD: unchanged
Naproxen	Bioavailability:95% Onset of action:30–60 min	Time to peak: tablets, naproxen:2-4h Tablets, naproxen sodium:1-2h Suspension:1-4h Protein binding:>99%, albumin; Vd:0.16 L/kg Duration:<12h	Hepatic: 6-0-desmethyl naproxen; parent drug, desmethyl metabolite, further metabolism to acylglucuronide conjugated metabolites	Urine:95% metabolites; feces:≤3% Half-life:12–17h; CrCl 30–60:15–21h
Ketorolac	PO: well absorbed, fatty meal decreased 1h; IM: rapid, complete Bioavailability: PO, IM:100% Onset of action: 30 min	Time to peak PO:45 min; IM:30–45 min; IV:1-3 min Protein binding:99%; Vd: PO, IM:0.17 ± 0.04 L/kg; IV:0.21 ± 0.04 L/kg Peak effect:2-3h Duration:4-6h	Hepatic: hydroxylation, glucuronide conjugation; OAT1/3 substrate	Urine:92%, 60% unchanged drug; feces:6% Half-life:5h(2-9h); S-enantiomer:2.5 h (biologically active); R-enantiomer:5h; elderly: increased 30%–50%; Scr 1.9-5 mg/dL:11h(4–19h); dialysis:14h(8–40h)

(continued on next page)

Table 1
(continued)

Drug	Absorption	Distribution	Metabolism	Excretion
Celecoxib	Capsule: prolonged PO solution: rapid Bioavailability: PO solution:144% (relative to capsule)	Time to peak: capsule:3h; PO solution:1h Protein binding:97%, albumin; alpha1-acid glycoprotein; Vd: capsule:400L; PO solution:288–743L	Hepatic: CYP2C9; inactive metabolites (alcohol, carboxylic acid, glucuronide conjugate); major CYP2C9 substrate	Urine:27% metabolites, <3% unchanged drug; feces:57% metabolites, <3% unchanged drug Half-life: capsule:11h (fasting); PO solution:1h; CrCl 35–60: AUC decreased 40%; Child-Pugh class A: AUC increased 40%; Child-Pugh class B: AUC increased 180%; Elderly: capsule: Cmax increased 40%, AUC increased 50%; capsule: AUC increased 40% in Black patients compared with White patients.
Hydrocodone	N/A	Time to peak:1h	Hepatic: O-demethylation via CYP2D6 to hydromorphone (>100x higher binding affinity for mu-opioid receptor than hydrocodone), N-demethylation via CYP3A4 to norhydrocodone, 40% metabolism via non-CYP pathways (6-ketosteroid reduction to 6-alpha-hydrocol, 6-beta-hydrocol), fecal, biliary, intestinal, renal	Urine:26% dose in 72h, 12% unchanged drug, 5% norhydrocodone, 4% conjugated hydrocodone, 3% 6-hydrocodol, 0.21% conjugated 6-hydromorphol Half-life:4h

OxyCODONE	Bioavailability: IR:60%–87% Onset of action: IR:10–15 min	Time to peak: IR:1.2-2h Protein binding:38%–45%; Vd:2.6 L/kg: distributed to skeletal muscle, liver, intestinal tract, lungs, spleen, brain Peak effect: IR:0.5-1h Duration: IR:3-6h	Hepatic: CYP3A4 to noroxycodone (weak analgesic), noroxymorphone, alpha- and beta-noroxycodol. CYP2D6 metabolism to oxymorphone (analgesic; <15% plasma concentrations), alpha- and beta-oxymorphol; major CYP3A4 substrate	Urine:10% parent, 65% active metabolites (23% noroxycodone, 10% oxymorphone, 14% noroxymorphone), ≤18% reduced metabolites Half-life: IR:3.2-4h; CrCl<60: increased 1h, Cmax 50%, AUC 60%; mild-moderate hepatic impairment increased 2.3 h, Cmax 50%, AUC 95%
Hydromorphone	PO: rapidly absorbed; extensive first-pass effect; IM: variable and delayed Bioavailability: PO, IR:24% Onset of action: IR: PO:15–30 min	Time to peak: IR:≤1h Protein binding:8%–19%; Vd:4 L/kg Peak effect:30–60 min IV:5 min; Peak effect:10–20 min Duration: IR: PO, IV:3-4h; suppository may provide longer effect	Hepatic: glucuronidation, inactive metabolites, >95% metabolized to hydromorphone-3-glucuronide, <5% 6-hydroxy reduction metabolites	Urine: glucuronide conjugates, 7% unchanged drug excreted in urine; feces:1% Half-life: IR:2-3h Renal impairment: IR: CrCl 40–60: Cmax and AUC increased 2x; CrCl<30: Cmax and AUC increased 3x Hepatic impairment (Child-Pugh class B): Cmax and AUC increased 4x IR: (female) 25% higher Cmax
Fentanyl	Onset of action: IM:7-8 min IV: almost immediate	Protein binding:79%–87%, alpha-1 acid glycoprotein, albumin, erythrocytes; Vd:4-6 L/kg Duration: IM:1-2h; IV:0.5-1h respiratory depressant > analgesic	Hepatic: CYP3A4 via N-dealkylation to norfentanyl and hydroxylation to inactive metabolites; major CYP3A4 substrate	Urine:75% metabolites, 7%–10% unchanged drug; feces:9% Half-life: continuous infusion:2-4h, increased by duration
Tapentadol	Rapid, complete Bioavailability:32%	Time to peak IR:1.25 h Protein binding:20%; Vd: IV:442–638L	Hepatic: phase 2 glucuronidation to tapentadol-O-glucuronide; minimal phase 1 oxidative metabolism via CYP2C9, CYP2C19, CYP2D6; all inactive metabolites	Urine:99%, 70% conjugated metabolites, 3% unchanged drug Half-life: IR:4h

(continued on next page)

Table 1
(continued)

Drug	Absorption	Distribution	Metabolism	Excretion
Tramadol	Bioavailability: IR:75% Onset of action: IR:<1h; Peak effect:2–3h	Time to peak: IR:2h; active metabolite (M1: O-desmethyl tramadol):3h; M1:5–15h Protein binding:20%; Vd: IV:2.6 L/kg (males); 2.9 L/kg (females) IR:(female) 12% higher Cmax, 35% higher AUC	Hepatic: prodrug, demethylation via CYP3A4, CYP2D6, glucuronidation, sulfation; M1 formed via CYP2D6; major CYP2D6 and CYP3A4 substrates; Poor metabolizers: M1 40% lower	Urine:30% unchanged drug, 60% metabolites Half-life: IR:6.3 ± 1.4 h; M1:7.4 ± 1.4 h; increased in elderly
Methadone	Bioavailability: PO:36%–100% Onset of action: PO:0.5-1h; IV:10–20 min	Time to peak:1–7.5 h Protein binding:80%–90%, alpha-1 acid glycoprotein; Vd:1-8 L/kg Peak effect:IV:1-2h; PO:3-5 d; IV:10-20 min; Duration: PO:4-8h (single dose); 8–12h (repeat dose)	Hepatic: N-demethylation via CYP3A4, CYP2B6, CYP2C19, CYP2C9, CYP2D6	Urine:<10% unchanged drug; increased with urine pH < 6; persists in liver and other tissues Half-life:8–59h; increased with alkaline pH, auto-induction of metabolism
Buprenorphine	IR: IM:30%–40% Ingestion of liquids decrease systemic exposure from buccal film by 23%–37% Bioavailability: buccal film: 46%–65%; IR IM:70% Onset of action: IR: IM:≥15 min	Time to peak: buccal film:2.5-3h; steady state achieved 4–6 mo Protein binding:96%, alpha- and beta globulin; Vd:218–806L Peak effect:1h Duration: IR IM:≥6h	Hepatic: N-dealkylation via CYP3A4 to norbuprenorphine, lesser extent glucuronidation by UGT1A1, UGT1A3 and 2B7 to buprenorphine 3-O-glucuronide; extensive first-pass effect; major CYP3A4 substrate	Urine:27%–30%, 1% unchanged drug, 9.4% conjugated drug, 2.7% norbuprenorphine, 11% conjugated norbuprenorphine; feces:70%, 33% unchanged drug, 5% conjugated drug, 21% norbuprenorphine, 2% conjugated norbuprenorphine Half-life: buccal film:27.6 ± 11.2 h; IV:2.2 h (1.2–7.2 h); 8.6-32.1 h for doses 0.3–16 mg

Naltrexone	PO: almost complete Bioavailability: PO:5%–40%	Time to peak: PO:60 min; IM: biphasic:2h (first peak), 2–3 d (second peak) Protein binding:21%; Vd:1350L Duration: PO: 50 mg:24h; 100 mg:48h; 150 mg:72h; IM:4 wk	Hepatic: noncytochrome-mediated dehydrogenase conversion to 6-beta-naltrexol and minor metabolites, forms glucuronide conjugates	Urine: metabolites and unchanged drug Half-life: PO:4h; 6-beta-naltrexol:13h; IM: parent and 6-beta-naltrexol:5–10 d
Gabapentin	Variable, proximal small bowel, saturable process; inversely dose-dependent Bioavailability: IR: 900 mg/day:60% 1,200 mg/day:47% 2,400 mg/day:34% 3,600 mg/day:33% 4,800 mg/day:27%	Time to peak: IR:2-4h; ER:8h Protein binding:<3%; Vd:58±6L	Not metabolized; OCT2 substrate	Urine: unchanged drug Half-life:5-7h; CrCl<30:52h; Anuric:132h Dialysis:3.8 h
Pregabalin	ER:(fasting): AUC decreased 30% Bioavailability:≥90% Onset of action:<1 wk	Time to peak: IR:(fasting):<1.5 h; (food):3h ER:(food):8h(5–12h) Protein binding:0%; Vd:0.5 L/kg	Not metabolized	Urine:90% unchanged drug, minor metabolites Half-life:6.3 h
Duloxetine	Well absorbed, (food): decreases AUC 10% Bioavailability: smokers: decreased 33%	Time to peak:5-6h; (food): delays 1.7-4h Protein binding:>90%; albumin, alpha1-acid glycoprotein; Vd:1,640L	Hepatic: CYP1A2, CYP2D6; multiple inactive metabolites	Urine:70%; <1% unchanged drug; feces:20% Half-life:12h(8–22h); elderly (female):4h longer
Amitriptyline	Rapid, well absorbed Bioavailability:43%–46%	Time to peak:2-5h Protein binding:>90%; Vd:18–22 L/kg	Hepatic: rapid demethylation to nortriptyline (active), hydroxy derivatives, conjugated derivatives; major CYP2D6 substrate	Urine: glucuronide or sulfate conjugate metabolites; Feces: small amounts Half-life:13–36h

(continued on next page)

Table 1
(continued)

Drug	Absorption	Distribution	Metabolism	Excretion
Ketamine	Bioavailability: PO:20%–30%; IM:93% Onset of action: PO:<30 min 4 mg/kg/dose:12.9 ± 1.9 min 6 mg/kg/dose:10.4 ± 2.9 min 8 mg/kg/dose:9.5 ± 1.9 min	Time to peak: PO:30 min; IM:5–30 min Protein binding:27%; Vd:2.1–3.1 L/kg Duration:15–30 min; recovery:3–4h	Hepatic: metabolite I: N-dealkylation to norketamine; metabolites III and IV: hydroxylation of cyclohexone ring, conjugation with glucuronic acid; metabolite II: dehydration of hydroxylated metabolites to cyclohexene derivative; norketamine 33% the potency of parent compound; major CYP2B6 and CYP3A4 substrates PO: norketamine concentrations increased	Urine:91%; feces:3% Half-life: alpha:10–15 min; beta:2.5 h
Cyclobenzaprine	Bioavailability:33%–55% Onset of action: IR:<1h	Time to peak: IR:4h Duration: IR:12–24h	Hepatic: CYP3A4, 1A2, 2D6; enterohepatic recirculation	Urine: glucuronide metabolites; feces: unchanged drug Half-life: IR:18h; hepatic impairment:46h (22–188h) Elderly:(male) AUC increased 2.4x; (female) AUC increased 1.2x
Tizanidine	Tablets (food): increased 30%; capsules (food): increased 10% Bioavailability:40%	Time to peak: capsule, tablet (fasting):1h; capsule (food):3-4h, tablet (food):1.5 h Protein binding:30%; Vd: IV:2.4 L/kg Duration:3-6h	Hepatic: CYP1A2 to inactive metabolites; major CYP1A2 substrate	Urine:60%; feces:20% Half-life:2.5 h

Methocarbamol	Onset of action: PO:30 min	Time to peak: PO:1-2h Protein binding:46%–60%	Hepatic: dealkylation, hydroxylation	Urine: metabolites Severe renal impairment: clearance decreased 40%; hepatic impairment: clearance decreased 70% Half-life:1-2h; cirrhosis: increased 3x
Diazepam	PO: well absorbed >90%; (fatty food): delayed and decreased; PR: well absorbed Bioavailability: PO:>90%; IM:>90%; PR:90%	Time to peak: PO:15min-2.5 h (fasting):1.25 h; (food):2.5 h; IM:1h (0.25-2h); IV:1 min; PR:1.5 h Protein binding:98%; Vd: PO; IV; PR:1.1 L/kg (0.6–1.8) Duration:>40h	Hepatic: N-demethylated by CYP3A4 and 2C19 to active metabolite N-desmethyldiazepam, hydroxylated by CYP3A4 to active metabolite temazepam, N-desmethyldiazepam and temazepam metabolized to oxazepam, temazepam and oxazepam eliminated by glucuronidation; major CYP2C19 and CYP3A4 substrates	Urine: glucuronide conjugates Half-life: accumulates with multi-dosing PO: parent:44–48h; desmethyldiazepam: 100h; IM: parent:60–72h; desmethyldiazepam: 152–174h IV: parent:33–45h; desmethyldiazepam: 87h PR: parent:45–46h; desmethyldiazepam: 71–99h Mild and moderate cirrhosis:>500h; hepatic fibrosis:90h (66–104h); chronic active hepatitis:60h(26–76h); acute viral hepatitis:74h (49–129h) Half-life increased 1h each year of age
HydrOXYzine	PO: rapid Onset of action: PO:15–30 min	Time to peak: PO:2h Vd:16±3 L/kg; elderly:23 L/kg; hepatic dysfunction:23 L/kg Duration: pruritus suppression:1–12h	Hepatic: multiple metabolites, including cetirizine	Urine: cetirizine renally eliminated Half-life:20h; elderly:29h; hepatic impairment:37h

(continued on next page)

Table 1
(continued)

Drug	Absorption	Distribution	Metabolism	Excretion
Ascorbic acid (vitamin C)	PO: intestine, saturable process; dose-dependent 30–180 mg/day = 70–90%, >1,000 mg/day≤50% Bioavailability: PO: 200 mg = 100%; 1250 mg = 33%	N/A	Hepatic: reversibly oxidized to DHA, ascorbic acid and DHA are active	Urine: serum concentrations >80 mg/day excreted Half-life:10h; biological:8–40 d

Abbreviations: AUC, area under the curve; Cmax, maximum serum concentration; CrCl, creatinine clearance (mL/min); DHA, dehydroascorbic acid; ER, extended release; ESRD, end stage renal disease; GI, gastrointestinal; h, hours; IM, intramuscular; IR, immediate release; IV, intravenous; min, minutes; N/A, not applicable; NAPQI, N-acetyl-p-benzoquinone imine; PO, by mouth; PR, rectal; sec, seconds; SubQ, subcutaneous; Vd, volume of distribution.

he burn patient transitions to the hypermetabolic burn state, blood flow increases to the kidneys, resulting in increased drug excretion, measured using the CrCl. Increased CrCl may require higher doses of drugs or more frequent dosing intervals to maintain therapeutic plasma drug concentrations. Drug excretion may also occur through areas of burned tissue. Fluids, proteins, and drugs may be lost through these compromised skin barriers.[21,22]

PHARMACOLOGIC MANAGEMENT

The source of pain must first be identified as nociceptive, neuropathic, or nociplastic to direct appropriate pharmacologic management. The appropriate pharmacologic management should be tailored to each patient depending on individual patient-related factors. This includes knowledge and understanding of pharmacokinetics, pharmacodynamics, pharmacoeconomics, pharmacogenomics, and pharmacotherapeutics.[21,23] These factors are influenced by a patient's genome, age, sex, race, allergies, diet, comorbidities, renal function, hepatic function, available drug routes, drug interactions, adverse effects, contraindications to use, and pathophysiologic burn phases following burn injuries. Combination therapy increases efficacy and reduces toxicity by offering a multimodal approach to burn-related pain by targeting different receptors in the PNS and CNS. Receptors may be targeted by drugs through systemic, regional, local, and/or topical routes of administration. It is important to incorporate physical therapy, occupational therapy, and psychological counseling early into the multimodal approach. Surgical etiologies of pain related to direct nerve injury or compression should be identified early to avoid unnecessary exposure to pharmacologic agents. If burn-related pain is amenable to surgical interventions, these interventions should be considered early.[6]

Shared decision-making is essential to tailor patient expectations and provide early education to avoid developing chronic pain. Frequent follow ups should be considered to strengthen the therapeutic alliance between the patient and management team. Realistic goals for pain and function must be established, including the possible inability to achieve "0" pain severity. Discussions should initially include the importance of adherence to management, scheduling doses to stay ahead of pain symptoms, then transitioning to as needed dosing, avoiding extended-release formulations, using the minimum effective dose for the shortest interval possible, risks of developing chronic pain secondary to CNS changes from prolonged use of drugs, tapering drugs to avoid abrupt discontinuation, how therapy will be discontinued if benefits do not outweigh risks.

ROUTES OF ADMINISTRATION
Systemic

Systemic administration affects the entire body by releasing the drug into the circulatory system for distribution to receptors. This may be beneficial for large %TBSA burns; however, smaller burns may be more amenable to more localized management. Systemic administration has the potential to increase drug exposure throughout the entire body, resulting in lower drug concentrations at target receptors and higher risks of adverse effects by binding off-target receptors. Systemic routes of administration include oral, intravenous, rectal, and transdermal patches. Transdermal and topical drugs should be avoided over areas of burned tissue due to unpredictable absorption, risks of higher systemic drug exposure, and adverse effects.

Regional

Regional administration may be achieved with epidural or targeted nerve analgesia. Epidural analgesia distributes the drug in the epidural space to provide full pain blockade below the level of administration in the CNS. Advantages of regional anesthesia include administration of higher drug concentrations with less systemic toxicity, while disadvantages may include blockade with temporary loss of signaling to potentially unburned tissues.[24] Nerve blocks may provide intermittent or continuous pain relief by targeting single or groups of sensory nerves along anatomic nerve distributions. Nerve blocks can effectively be administered prior to performing dressing changes and decrease opioid requirements.[25,26] Commonly used medications are lidocaine, ropivacaine, and bupivacaine. Lidocaine and ropivacaine have more rapid onsets of action, while bupivacaine has a longer duration of action.[27] For burns to the upper extremity, brachial plexus blocks may achieve successful neural blockade. Axillary, infraclavicular, and supraclavicular blocks may be used for hand burns, while the interscalene block is used for shoulder and upper arm burns. Lower extremity nerve blocks may be performed targeting the lumbar plexus, sciatic, lateral femoral cutaneous, fascia iliaca, femoral, obturator, genicular, popliteal, and saphenous nerves.[28]

Local and Topical

Local and topical administration provides an anesthetic or analgesic directly to the area of pain.

Tumescent analgesia is a local method of infiltrating a dilute concentration of solution of anesthetic, commonly lidocaine, combined with epinephrine, sodium bicarbonate and other adjunctive drugs into the subcutaneous or subdermal layer of the skin graft donor site using a spinal needle until the tissue becomes firm and tense. Topical formulations of anesthetics can be used as alternatives to injections or to reduce the pain, needle anxiety and edema at sites prior to injections. Commonly used topical formulations include various combinations with the active drug lidocaine. Local and topical routes of administration can allow patients to undergo minor procedures without the need of general anesthesia.

ACUTE MANAGEMENT

A pharmacologic regimen should consist of using a stepwise approach with base management and adjuncts tailored to each patient for burn-related acute nociceptive and/or neuropathic pain (Fig. 2). Drug pharmacokinetics and pharmacodynamics are important considerations for acute

burn-related pain (see Table 1).[21] Initially, patients should be started at lower drug doses using multimodal targeted management, then titrate doses and add drugs to achieve burn-related pain relief (Table 2).

Acute Nociceptive and Neuropathic Pain

Certain drugs may be beneficial as base management and as adjuncts for both acute nociceptive and neuropathic pain. Both types of acute pain may benefit from vitamin C and an opioid or mixed opioid. Vitamin C administration may be beneficial therapy for acute and chronic burn-related pain, with a low risk-to-benefit trade-off that may provide additional advantages for patients, such as enhanced wound healing.[11]

No evidence exists regarding the superiority of one opioid over another. Opioids should be administered for burn-related acute moderate to severe nociceptive or neuropathic pain in combination with multimodal management.[29] Patients who have not taken an opioid for 1 to 2 weeks should be considered opioid naïve. Nonopioid analgesics

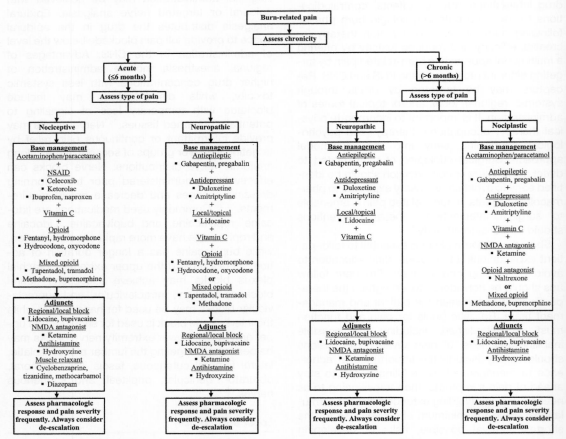

Fig. 2. Multimodal Pharmacologic Management Algorithm of Burn-related Pain. NMDA, N-methyl-D-aspartate receptor; NSAID, nonsteroidal anti-inflammatory drug.

Table 2
Drugs, adult dosing, contraindications and clinical pearls for pain management

Drug/MOA	Dosing	Renal Impairment	Hepatic Impairment	Contraindications	Clinical Pearls
Acetaminophen/ paracetamol *MOA:* Not fully elucidated, activation of descending serotonergic inhibitory pathways in the CNS. Interactions with other nociceptive systems	*Nociceptive (mild-moderate)* PO:325–650 mg q4h-q6h PRN or 1g q6h PRN; max: 4 g/day IV:≥50 kg:650 mg q4h or 1g q6h; max single dose:1 g/dose; max:4 g/day <50 kg:12.5 mg/kg q4h or 15 mg/kg q6h; max single dose:15 mg/kg/ dose (≤750 mg/dose); max:≤3.75 g/day PR:325–650 mg q4h-q6h; max:3.9 g/day	*Mild-severe impairment:* no adjustment IV: q6h-q8h *Hemodialysis, intermittent; peritoneal dialysis:* no *CRRT; PIRRT:* no adjustment	*Child-Turcotte-Pugh class A Active alcohol use:* max:2 g/day *No active alcohol use:* ≤14 d: no adjustment >14 d: max:3 g/day *Child-Turcotte-Pugh class B: Active alcohol use:* max:2 g/day *No active alcohol use:* ≤14 d: max:3 g/day >14 d: max:2 g/day *Child-Turcotte-Pugh class C:* IV: avoid; PO, PR: max:2 g/day	Hypersensitivity; severe hepatic impairment; severe active liver disease	Risk of medication errors; hepatotoxicity; acute liver failure, resulting in liver transplant and death
Ibuprofen (NSAID) *MOA:* Reversibly inhibits COX-1 and COX-2 enzymes, decreases prostaglandin precursors; inhibits chemotaxis, alters lymphocyte activity, inhibits neutrophil aggregation/ activation, and decreases proinflammatory cytokine levels	*Nociceptive (mild-moderate) Acute:* IV, PO: initially schedule doses 200–400 mg q4h-q6h PRN or 600–800 mg q6h-q8h PRN; max:3.2 g/day *Chronic:* max:2.4 g/day	*CrCl 30–60:* no adjustment; avoid if hypovolemic, hypotensive, elderly, concurrent nephrotoxic drugs *CrCl ≤30:* avoid *Hemodialysis, intermittent; peritoneal dialysis:* no adjustment *CRRT; PIRRT:* avoid	No adjustment	All NSAIDs (Hypersensitivity; history of asthma or urticaria with aspirin; CABG surgery; bleeding; thrombocytopenia; coagulation defects; necrotizing enterocolitis; renal dysfunction)	All NSAIDs (Cardiovascular thrombotic events, MI, stroke; GI events including bleeding, ulceration, perforation of stomach or intestines), greatest risk with SNRI/SSRI and corticosteroids; hypertension; renal impairment; take with food

(continued on next page)

Table 2
(continued)

Drug/MOA	Dosing	Renal Impairment	Hepatic Impairment	Contraindications	Clinical Pearls
Naproxen (NSAID) *MOA:* Same for all NSAIDs	*Nociceptive (mild-moderate)* *Acute:* PO: IR:500 mg once, followed by 250–500 mg q12 h PRN or 250 mg q6h-q8h PRN; max:1.25 g day 1, then 1 g/day. Initially schedule doses ER:1 g/day; increase to 1.5 g/day for acute pain, then reduce to max 1 g/day	*CrCl 30–60:* no adjustment. Avoid if hypovolemic, hypotensive, elderly, concurrent nephrotoxic drugs *CrCl ≤30:* avoid *Hemodialysis, intermittent; peritoneal dialysis; CRRT; PIRRT:* avoid *AKI:* discontinue	No adjustment	Same for all NSAIDs	Same for all NSAIDs
Ketorolac (NSAID) *MOA:* Same for all NSAIDs	*Nociceptive (moderate-severe)* *Acute* Max duration:5 d Weight ≥50 kg and age <65 y: IV:30 mg single dose or 15–30 mg q6h PRN; max:120 mg/day IM:30–60 mg single dose or 10–30 mg q4h-q6h PRN; max:120 mg/day PO:10 mg q4h-q6h PRN; max:40 mg/day Weight <50 kg or age ≥65 y: IV:15 mg as single dose or 15 mg q6h PRN; max dose:60 mg/day IM:30 mg single dose or 10–15 mg q4h-q6h PRN; max:60 mg/day PO:10 mg q4h-q6h PRN; max:40 mg/day	*eGFR 30–60:* IM, IV:7.5–15 mg q6h; avoid if hypovolemic, hypotensive, elderly, concurrent nephrotoxic drugs PO:10 mg q4h-q6h PRN; max:40 mg/day *eGFR ≤30:* IM, IV, PO: avoid *Hemodialysis, intermittent; peritoneal dialysis; CRRT; PIRRT:* avoid	No adjustment	Same for all NSAIDs; advanced renal disease or risk for renal failure; prophylactic analgesic before major surgery; suspected or confirmed cerebrovascular bleeding, hemorrhagic diathesis, incomplete hemostasis, high risk of bleeding; aspirin, NSAIDs, probenecid, pentoxifylline; epidural or intrathecal administration	Same for all NSAIDs; max duration 5 d; PO only indicated as continuation of IV/IM; renal failure; liver failure; special populations: dosage should be adjusted ≥65 y of age, <50 kg, elevated SCr

Celecoxib (NSAID) MOA: Inhibits prostaglandin synthesis by decreasing activity of enzyme, COX-2, results in decreased formation of prostaglandin precursors; does not inhibit COX-1	Nociceptive (mild-moderate) Acute PO: initial:400 mg, followed by 200 mg 12h on day 1; thereafter, 200 mg BID PRN or scheduled; max:400 mg/day	CrCl 30–60: no adjustment. Avoid if hypovolemic, hypotensive, elderly, concurrent nephrotoxic drugs CrCl ≤30: avoid Hemodialysis, intermittent; peritoneal dialysis; CRRT; PIRRT: avoid AKI: discontinue	Child-Pugh class B: reduce dose 50% Child-Pugh class C: avoid Abnormal LFTs: discontinue	Hypersensitivity sulfonamides, aspirin, NSAIDs; history of asthma or urticaria with aspirin; CABG surgery	Cardiovascular thrombotic events, MI, stroke; GI events including bleeding, ulceration, perforation of the stomach or intestines (lowest risk NSAID); Avoid with sulfa allergy
Hydrocodone (opioid) Class: phenanthrene MOA: Binds to opiate receptors in the CNS, altering the perception of and response to pain; suppresses cough in medullary center; produces generalized CNS depression	Nociceptive, neuropathic (moderate-severe) Acute: PO:5–10 mg q4h-q6h PRN Discontinuation or tapering of therapy: Initial tapers range from 10%/week or 25%–50% reduction every few days. Withdrawal symptoms, consider slowing the taper schedule; pausing the taper and restarting when the patient is ready, and/or coadministration of an alpha-2 agonist to blunt autonomic withdrawal symptoms	No adjustment	No adjustment	All opioids (Hypersensitivity; significant respiratory depression; acute or severe bronchial asthma in an unmonitored setting or absence of resuscitative equipment; GI obstruction, including paralytic ileus)	All opioids (Addiction, abuse, and misuse; life-threatening respiratory depression; neonatal opioid withdrawal syndrome; risks from concomitant use with benzodiazepines or other CNS depressants; medication errors)

(continued on next page)

Table 2
(continued)

Drug/MOA	Dosing	Renal Impairment	Hepatic Impairment	Contraindications	Clinical Pearls
OxyCODONE (opioid) Class: phenanthrene *MOA:* Same for all opioids	*Nociceptive, neuropathic (moderate-severe)* *Opioid-naive* *Acute:* PO: IR: initial:5 mg q4h-q6h PRN; 5–15 mg q4h-q6h PRN; max:30 mg/day *Chronic:* PO: IR: initial:2.5–10 mg q4h-q6h PRN; maintenance:5–15 mg q4h-q6h PRN or scheduled. Increase in increments of 25%–50% of daily dose *Opioid-tolerant* *Acute:* PO: IR: initial:10 mg q4h PRN. Doses ≥33 mg/day add no benefits	*CrCl 30–60:* IR: PO: initial:50%–75% dose q6h *CrCl <30; hemodialysis, intermittent; peritoneal dialysis:* IR: PO: initial:50% dose q8h *CRRT, PIRRT* IR: PO: initial:50% of dose q6h	IR:33%–50% dose, consider extending q6h-q12 h	Same for all opioids	Same for all opioids, risk of overdose with CYP3A4 inhibitors or discontinuing CYP3A4 inducers
Hydromorphone (opioid) Class: phenanthrene *MOA:* Same for all opioids	*Nociceptive, neuropathic (moderate-severe)* *Opioid-naive* *Acute:* PO: IR: initial:1-2 mg q4h-q6h PRN; 1-4 mg q4h-q6h PRN; Outpatient moderate max:8 mg/day; severe max:12 mg/day IV: Intermittent dosing: initial:0.2–0.5 mg q2h-q4h PRN; 0.2-1 mg q2h-q4h PRN	IV, PO: *CrCl 30–60:* initial:50% dose *CrCl <30:* IR: initial:25% dose; extend dosing interval 25%–50% *Hemodialysis, intermittent; peritoneal dialysis:* IR: initial:25% dose; extend dosing interval 25%–50% *CRRT, PIRRT:* initial:25%–50% dose; extend	*Mild-severe impairment:* IV, PO: initial: 25%–50% dose	Same for all opioids	Same for all opioids

	PCA: must have capacity to press button to titrate. Initiate after pain controlled Concentration:0.2 mg/mL Demand:0.1–0.3 mg Basal: avoid in opioid-naive Lockout interval:10–20 min Max cumulative:6 mg q4h Rescue bolus:0.1–0.3 mg *Chronic:* PO: IR: initial:1–2 mg q2h-q3h PRN or scheduled; 1-4 mg q2h-q3h PRN or scheduled. Increase in increments of 25%–50% of daily dose. Dosages ≥12.5 mg/day add no benefits			dosing interval 25%–50%	
Fentanyl (opioid) Class: phenylpiperidine *MOA:* Binds with stereospecific receptors at many sites within the CNS, increases pain threshold, alters pain reception, inhibits ascending pain pathways	*Nociceptive, neuropathic (moderate-severe)* Opioid-naive Acute, PCA: Concentration:10mcg/mL Demand:5–20mcg Basal: avoid in opioid-naive Lockout interval:5–10 min Max cumulative:300mcg q4h Rescue bolus:5–20mcg	No adjustment	No adjustment	Same for all opioids	Same for all opioids, CYP3A4 inhibitors increase fentanyl concentrations; medication errors when converting between formulations; preferred opioid for severe kidney or hepatic dysfunction

(continued on next page)

Table 2
(continued)

Drug/MOA	Dosing	Renal Impairment	Hepatic Impairment	Contraindications	Clinical Pearls
	Acute severe: IV: Intermittent: Loading dose:25–100mcg or 1-2mcg/kg; Maintenance:25–50mcg or 0.35–0.5mcg/kg q30min-q60 min PRN Continuous infusion: Initial:25–50mcg/h; titrate q30min-q60 min; 50–300mcg/h *BMI ≥30:* IV: use adjusted body weight for initial weight-based calculations				
Tapentadol (mixed opioid) *MOA:* Binds µ-opiate receptors in CNS causing inhibition of ascending pain pathways, altering perception and response to pain; inhibits the reuptake of norepinephrine, which modifies ascending pain pathways	*Nociceptive, neuropathic (moderate-severe)* Acute: PO: IR: day 1:50–100 mg q4h-q6h PRN; may administer second dose ≥1h after the first dose; max:700 mg/day; day ≥2:50–100 mg q4h-q6h PRN; max:600 mg/day	*CrCl <30:* avoid	*Child-Pugh class B:* IR: initial:50 mg q8h; max:150 mg/day *Child-Pugh class C:* avoid	Same for all opioids, concomitant use or <14 d following MAOI	Same for all opioids, risk of seizures; risk of serotonin syndrome; lower risk of GI effects compared to other opioids

| Tramadol (mixed opioid) *MOA:* Prodrug, active metabolite (M1) binds μ-opiate receptors in the CNS causing inhibition of ascending pain pathways, altering perception and response to pain; inhibits reuptake of norepinephrine and serotonin, neurotransmitters involved in descending inhibitory pain pathway responsible for pain relief | *Nociceptive, neuropathic (moderate-severe)* *Acute:* PO: IR: initial:50 mg q4h-q6h PRN; for rapid onset may consider initial dose 50–100 mg q4h-q6h; 25–50 mg TID; then increase 50–100 mg q4h-q6h PRN *Chronic (alternative agent):* not preferred for chronic noncancer pain *Opioid-naive:* PO: IR: initial:100 mg daily, titrate 100 mg/day q5days PRN; max:400 mg/day | *CrCl <30:* IR: increase dosing interval to q12 h; max:200 mg/day. *Hemodialysis, intermittent; peritoneal dialysis:* IR:25 mg BID; max:200 mg/day | Reduced hepatic metabolism = ineffective pain control *Liver cirrhosis* *Child-Turcotte-Pugh class A:* initial: 50 mg q8h PRN; may increase to q6h; max:200 mg/day *Child-Turcotte-Pugh class B:* initial: 25 mg q8h-q12 h PRN; max: 100 mg/day in 2–3 doses *Child-Turcotte-Pugh class C:* avoid *Chronic pain:* avoid *Worsening hepatic function, acute:* discontinue, resume once LFTs have stabilized or returned to baseline | Same for all opioids; ages <12 y; concomitant use or <14 d following MAOI | Same for all opioids; ultra-rapid metabolism from CYP2D6 polymorphism; interactions with drugs affecting CYP450 isoenzymes 3A4 inducers, 3A4 inhibitors, 2D6 inhibitors; risk of seizures; risk of serotonin syndrome; lower risk of GI effects compared to other opioids |
| Methadone (mixed opioid) Class: diphenylheptane *MOA:* Binds to opiate receptors in CNS, causing inhibition of ascending pain pathways, alters perception and response to pain; produces | *Nociceptive, neuropathic, nociplastic (moderate-severe)* *Acute:* PO:10–40 mg q6h-q12 h IV:2.5–10 mg q8h-q12 h *Opioid-naive* *Chronic:* PO:2.5–5 mg q8h-q12 h IM, IV:2.5–10 mg q8h-q12 h; increase 2.5 mg/dose q5days | PO, IV *CrCl >10:* no adjustment *CrCl ≤10:*50%–75% of dose *Hemodialysis, intermittent; Peritoneal dialysis; CRRT; PIRRT:* PO, IV: initial:50%–75% of dose | No adjustment | Same for all opioids | Same for all opioids; life-threatening QT prolongation; use with CYP3A4, 2B6, 2C19, 2C9, 2D6 inhibitors; decreased testosterone; risk of serotonin syndrome |

(continued on next page)

Table 2
(continued)

Drug/MOA	Dosing	Renal Impairment	Hepatic Impairment	Contraindications	Clinical Pearls
generalized CNS depression. N-methyl-D-aspartate (NMDA) receptor antagonis	*Opioid-tolerant* *Chronic:* max:40 mg/day				
Buprenorphine (mixed opioid) *MOA:* High-affinity binding to mu opiate receptors in the CNS; partial mu agonist and weak kappa antagonist activity. Due to it being a partial mu agonist, its analgesic effects plateau at higher doses and it then behaves like an antagonist	*Nociceptive, nociplastic (moderate-severe)* *Acute (moderate-severe):* IR: IM, IV: initial:0.3 mg q6h–q8h PRN; initial; max:0.3 mg; may repeat once 30–60 min *Chronic (moderate-severe):* Buccal film: titrate 150mcg q12 h, q4days; 600–900mcg doses following titration; max:900mcg q12 h. Oral burns, reduce starting and titration dose 50% *Opioid-naive initial:* buccal:75mcg daily or q12 h ≥ 4 d, then increase 150mcg q12 h *Opioid-tolerant* Daily dose <30 mg PO MME: initial: buccal:75mcg daily or q12 h Daily dose 30–89 mg PO MME: initial: buccal:150mcg q12 h	No adjustment	*Child-Pugh class C:* Buccal film: reduce dose 50% IR: IM, IV: no adjustment	Same for all opioids	Same for all opioids; accidental exposure (buccal film, transdermal patch); addiction, abuse, and misuse; life-threatening respiratory depression; risks from concomitant use with benzodiazepines or other CNS depressants; risk of serious harm or death with IV administration

Drug/MOA	Dosing	Renal adjustment	Hepatic adjustment	Adverse effects
	Daily dose 90–160 mg PO MME: initial: buccal: 300mcg q12 h Daily dose >160 mg PO MME: use alternate analgesic	No adjustment	Hypersensitivity; current physiologic opioid dependence, current use of opioid analgesics; acute opioid withdrawal; failure to pass naloxone challenge, positive urine screen for opioids	Acute withdrawal with higher doses
Naltrexone (opioid antagonist) *MOA:* Cyclopropyl derivative of oxymorphone; acts as a competitive antagonist at opioid receptor sites, showing the highest affinity for mu receptors	*Nociplastic (moderate-severe):* PO:4.5 mg daily (low-dose) *Pruritus:* Opioid-induced, associated with neuraxial opioid administration: PO:6 mg once; >6 mg may reverse analgesia Nonopioid-induced: PO:12.5–50 mg daily	No adjustment		
Gabapentin (antiepileptic) *MOA:* Does not bind to GABAA or GABAB receptors or influence degradation or uptake of GABA. Binds presynaptic voltage-gated calcium channels possessing the alpha-2-delta-1 subunit. May modulate release of excitatory neurotransmitters in nociception.	*Neuropathic, nociplastic:* Adequate trial ≥2 mo IR: PO: initial:100–300 mg TID, max:1.2 g TID ER: PO: initial:300 mg HS; max:3.6 g/day *Pruritus* IR: PO: initial:300 mg/day; max:1.8 g/day	IR: *CrCl >79:*3,600 mg/day *CrCl 50–79:*1,800 mg/day *CrCl 30–49:*50% reduction, 900 mg/day *CrCl 15–29:*75% reduction, 600 mg/day *CrCl <15:*90% reduction, 300 mg/day *Hemodialysis, intermittent:* 50% over 4h; Initial:100 mg TIW after hemodialysis; max:300 mg TIW *Peritoneal dialysis:* Initial:100 mg qod; max:300 mg/day *CRRT*	*Child-Turcotte-Pugh class B/C:* initial: ≤300 mg/day Progression from *Child-Turcotte-Pugh class A to B:* caution Progression to *Child-Turcotte-Pugh class B and C:* no adjustment	Somnolence; ataxia; peripheral edema; weight gain; diplopia; blurred vision; xerostomia

(continued on next page)

Table 2
(continued)

Drug/MOA	Dosing	Renal Impairment	Hepatic Impairment	Contraindications	Clinical Pearls
		CVVH; CVVHD; CVVHDF: initial:100 mg BID; max:300 mg BID *ER* *CrCl 30–59:600mg-1.8 g daily* *CrCl <30: avoid* *ESRD; peritoneal dialysis: avoid*			
Pregabalin (antiepileptic) *MOA:* Does not bind to GABA. Binds alpha-2-delta subunit of voltage-gated calcium channels within the CNS and modulates calcium influx at the nerve terminals, inhibits excitatory neurotransmitter release including glutamate, norepinephrine, serotonin, dopamine, substance P, calcitonin gene-related peptide. May affect descending noradrenergic, serotonergic pain transmission pathways from	*Neuropathic, nociplastic* IR: PO: initial:25–150 mg/day; increase 25–150 mg/day weekly to 300–600 mg/day in 2–3 doses *Pruritus* IR: PO: initial:75 mg BID; increase 150–300 mg/day in 2–3 doses	*Neuropathic* CrCl ≥60:300–600 mg/day CrCl 30–59:150–300 mg/day CrCl 15–29:75–150 mg/day CrCl <15:25–75 mg/day *Pruritus* CrCl ≥60:150–300 mg/day CrCl 30–59:75–150 mg/day CrCl 15–29:25–75 mg/day CrCl <15:25–50 mg/day *Hemodialysis, intermittent; peritoneal dialysis:* Initial:25 mg/day; max:75 mg/day *CRRT:* Initial:50 mg/day; max:300 mg/day *PIRRT:* PIRRT days: Initial:50 mg/day; max 300 mg/day, non-PIRRT days:75 mg/day	No adjustment	Hypersensitivity	Somnolence; ataxia; peripheral edema; weight gain; diplopia; blurred vision; xerostomia; euphoria

	Indication; Dosing	Renal Adjustment	Hepatic Adjustment	Contraindications	Adverse Effects / Warnings
brainstem to spinal cord					
Duloxetine (SNRI) *MOA:* Potent inhibitor of neuronal serotonin and norepinephrine reuptake, weak inhibitor of dopamine reuptake. No significant activity for muscarinic cholinergic, H1-histaminergic, or alpha2-adrenergic receptors. No MAO-inhibition	*Neuropathic, nociplastic Chronic musculoskeletal:* PO: initial:30 mg/day 1–2 wk, max:120 mg/day	*CrCl <30:* avoid; if necessary max:60 mg/day *Hemodialysis; Peritoneal dialysis:* avoid *CRRT; PIRRT:* refer to CrCl <30	Avoid	MAOIs concurrently or <14 d of discontinuing; <5 d of discontinuing duloxetine; initiation with linezolid or IV methylene blue	Suicidal thoughts and behavior in pediatric and young adults; hypertension; tachycardia; sexual dysfunction; xerostomia
Amitriptyline (TCA) *MOA:* Increases synaptic concentration of serotonin and/or norepinephrine in CNS by inhibition of reuptake by the presynaptic neuronal membrane pump	*Neuropathic, nociplastic Chronic:* PO: initial:10–25 mg HS; increase dose 10–25 mg at intervals ≥1 wk; max:150 mg/day, HS, or 2 doses	No adjustment	No adjustment; max:100 mg/day	Hypersensitivity; coadministration or <14 d of MAOIs; coadministration with cisapride; acute recovery phase following MI	Suicidal thoughts and behavior in pediatric and young adults; life-threatening QT prolongation; orthostatic hypotension, anticholinergic effects; avoid in elderly
Lidocaine *MOA:* Blocks initiation and conduction of nerve impulses by decreasing the neuronal membrane's permeability to sodium ions, results in inhibition of	*Nociceptive, neuropathic, nociplastic* Cutaneous infiltration: max:4.5 mg/kg/dose not to exceed 300 mg < 2h Cream: apply q6h-q8h PRN, max: 3 applications q24 h	No adjustment	No adjustment	Hypersensitivity; Adam-Stokes syndrome; Wolff-Parkinson-White syndrome; severe degrees of SA, AV, or intraventricular heart block; allergy to corn or corn-related	Arrhythmia

(continued on next page)

Table 2
(continued)

Drug/MOA	Dosing	Renal Impairment	Hepatic Impairment	Contraindications	Clinical Pearls
depolarization with resultant blockade of conduction	Gel: apply ≤ QID PRN; max:4.5 mg/kg, not to exceed 300 mg) Lotion: apply BID-QID Ointment: apply TID-QID; not to exceed 5g of ointment (equivalent to lidocaine base 250 mg) in a single application; maximum:20g of ointment/day (equivalent to lidocaine base 1,000 mg/day) Oral solution (2%):15 mL swished and spit q3h (max:4.5 mg/kg [300 mg/dose]; 8 doses/day) Oral solution (4%):1-5 mL (max:4.5 mg/kg [300 mg/dose] Patch (5%): apply for 12h. 1 patch/24h			products; traumatized mucosa; bacterial infection at application site; tuberculous or fungal lesions of skin vaccinia; varicella and acute herpes simplex	
Bupivacaine *MOA:* Blocks initiation and conduction of nerve impulses by decreasing the neuronal membrane's permeability to sodium ions, which	*Nociceptive, neuropathic, nociplastic* *Acute:* Peripheral nerve block:5 mL of 0.25%–0.5%; max:400 mg/day Sympathetic nerve block:20–50 mL of 0.25%	No adjustment	No adjustment	Hypersensitivity; obstetric paracervical block anesthesia; IV regional anesthesia (Bier block) (injection)	Risk of embolic effects resulting from inadvertent intravascular injection; arrhythmia

results in inhibition of depolarization with resultant blockade of conduction	Liposomal Regional analgesia: Interscalene brachial plexus nerve block: single dose:133 mg (10 mL); max:266 mg (20 mL)		
Ketamine (NMDA antagonist) *MOA:* Produces a cataleptic-like state dissociated from the surrounding environment by direct action on the cortex and limbic system. Noncompetitive NMDA receptor antagonist that blocks glutamate. Low doses produce analgesia, and modulate central sensitization, hyperalgesia and opioid tolerance. Reduces polysynaptic spinal reflexes.	*Nociceptive, neuropathic, nociplastic* *Acute:* Moderate-severe painful procedures, conditions that do not respond to standard analgesics IV: initial:0.25–0.5 mg/kg bolus; max:35 mg, followed by 0.05–0.25 mg/kg/h continuous infusion in longer duration of analgesia; titrate to:0.05-1 mg/kg/h; infusion duration:48–72h *Chronic:* PO: initial:0.5 mg/kg/day in 3–4 doses PRN; increase increments 5 mg/dose; max:800 mg/day *BMI 30–39:* use actual body weight for weight-based dosing *BMI ≥40:* use adjusted body weight or ideal body weight	No adjustment	No adjustment	Hypersensitivity; conditions which an increase in blood pressure would be hazardous; procedural sedation analgesia in emergency department; known or suspected schizophrenia	Hypertension; tachycardia; arrhythmia; laryngospasm; hallucinations; delirium; respiratory depression; genitourinary effects; drug dependence

(continued on next page)

Table 2
(continued)

Drug/MOA	Dosing	Renal Impairment	Hepatic Impairment	Contraindications	Clinical Pearls
Cyclobenzaprine (muscle relaxant) *MOA:* Centrally-acting skeletal muscle relaxant pharmacologically related to tricyclic antidepressants; reduces tonic somatic motor activity influencing both alpha and gamma motor neurons	*Muscle spasm:* temporarily or intermittently for a few days PO: IR: initial:5 mg TID scheduled or PRN; increase to 10 mg TID PRN; daily HS	No adjustment	*Moderate-severe impairment:* avoid	Hypersensitivity; during or <14 d of MAOIs; hyperthyroidism; heart failure; arrhythmias; heart block, conduction disturbances; acute recovery phase of MI	All muscle relaxants (sedation; dizziness; confusion); xerostomia
Tizanidine (muscle relaxant) *MOA:* Alpha2-adrenergic agonist which decreases spasticity by increasing presynaptic inhibition; effects greatest on polysynaptic pathways; overall reduces facilitation of spinal motor neurons	*Muscle spasm:* temporarily or intermittently for a few days PO: initial:4 mg q8h-q12 h PRN HS; max:24 mg/day	*CrCl <25:* initial:2 mg/day; increase 2 mg/day with minimum 1–4 d between increases *Hemodialysis, intermittent; peritoneal dialysis; CRRT; PIRRT* PO: initial:2 mg/day; increase 2 mg increments	*Impairment:* avoid	Hypersensitivity; concomitant therapy with potent CYP1A2 inhibitors	Same for all muscle relaxants; hypotension; xerostomia; weakness
Methocarbamol (muscle relaxant) *MOA:* Skeletal muscle relaxation by	*Muscle spasm:* temporarily or intermittently for a few days	No adjustment	No adjustment	Hypersensitivity; renal impairment (IV formulation)	MOA by sedation

general CNS depression	PO:1.5 g TID-QID for 2–3 d; max:8 g/day, then decrease dose ≤4.5 g/day; IM, IV: initial:1g q8h; max dose:3 g/day ≤3 consecutive days. May repeat after 48h drug-free interval		
Diazepam (muscle relaxant) MOA: Binds stereospecific benzodiazepine receptors on postsynaptic GABA neuron at several sites within the CNS, includes limbic system, reticular formation. Enhances inhibitory effect of GABA on neuronal excitability increasing neuronal membrane permeability to chloride ions. Results in hyperpolarization and stabilization. Selectively binds GABA-A receptors.	Muscle spasm: temporarily or intermittently for a few days PO: Initial:2 mg BID or 5 mg HS; increase gradually; max:60 mg/day	No adjustment _Severe impairment:_ avoid	Hypersensitivity; acute narrow-angle glaucoma; untreated open-angle glaucoma; PO: infants <6 mo of age, myasthenia gravis, severe respiratory impairment, severe hepatic impairment, sleep apnea syndrome Risks from concomitant use with opioids: profound sedation, respiratory depression, coma, and death; abuse, misuse, and addiction; dependence and withdrawal reactions; amnesia; Avoid in elderly

(continued on next page)

Table 2
(continued)

Drug/MOA	Dosing	Renal Impairment	Hepatic Impairment	Contraindications	Clinical Pearls
HydrOXYzine (antihistamine) *MOA:* Competes with histamine for H1-receptor sites on effector cells in the gastrointestinal tract, blood vessels, and respiratory tract. Possesses skeletal muscle relaxing, bronchodilator, antihistamine, antiemetic, analgesic properties. Activity at muscarinic, serotonergic (5HT2), dopaminergic receptors in the hippocampus, cerebral cortices, and brain may produce anxiolytic effects	*Pruritus, nociceptive, neuropathic:* PO:10–25 mg TID-QID PRN	*CrCl 10–49:*50% dose *CrCl <10:*25%–50% dose *Hemodialysis, intermittent; peritoneal dialysis:*25%–50% dose *CRRT, PIRRT:*50% dose	*Primary biliary cirrhosis:* dosing interval q24 h	Hypersensitivity to cetirizine or levocetirizine; early pregnancy; prolonged QT interval	Drowsiness; cognitive impairment; risk of QT prolongation; anticholinergic effects
Ascorbic acid (vitamin C) *MOA:* Essential water-soluble vitamin that acts as a cofactor and antioxidant. Electron donor used for collagen hydroxylation, carnitine biosynthesis,	*Nociceptive, neuropathic, nociplastic* PO, IM, IV:1-2g daily in 3 doses	No adjustment *Hemodialysis:* IV, PO:60–100 mg daily to prevent serious deficiency due to loss from dialysis	No adjustment	None	Oxalate nephropathy; nephrolithiasis

hormone/amino
acid biosynthesis.
Required for
connective tissue
synthesis, iron
absorption, storage

Abbreviations: AKI, acute kidney injury; BID, twice daily; CABG, coronary artery bypass graft; CNS, central nervous system; COX, cyclooxygenase; CrCl, creatinine clearance (mL/minute); CRRT, continuous renal replacement therapy; ER, extended release; ESRD, end stage renal disease; GFR, glomerular filtration rate; GI, gastrointestinal; h, hours; HS, at bedtime; IM, intramuscular; IR, immediate release; IV, intravenous; LFT, liver function tests; M1, active metabolite; MAOI, monoamine oxidase inhibitors; MI, myocardial infarction; min, minutes; MME, morphine milligram equivalents; MOA, mechanism of action; NMDA, N-methyl-D-aspartate receptor; NSAID, nonsteroidal anti-inflammatory drug; PCA, Patient-controlled analgesia; PIRRT, prolonged intermittent renal replacement therapy; PO, by mouth; PR, rectal; PRN, as needed; q, every; QID, 4 times daily; qod, every other day; sec, seconds; SNRI, serotonin norepinephrine reuptake inhibitors; SSRI, selective serotonin reuptake inhibitors; SubQ, subcutaneous; TCAs, tricyclic antidepressants; TID, 3 times daily; TIW, 3 times per week.

should be maximized, and the quantity prescribed should be limited to the expected duration of pain severe enough to require opioids. Long-acting formulations have not been found to be superior to short-acting formulations and should be avoided.[29] Early discussions should include OIH, including information on differentiating OIH symptoms from those of opioid tolerance and withdrawal.[30–32] Morphine is commonly avoided for burn-related pain secondary to a drug-induced histamine release that can further exacerbate pruritus.[33] Fentanyl may be used inpatient for pain. Its rapid onset, high-potency, and short duration of action make fentanyl a great drug for procedures and dressing changes in the burn unit.[34,35] Patients will need to be transitioned to an opioid that is available in an oral formulation prior to discharge if still requiring outpatient opioid management. Hydrocodone, oxycodone, and hydromorphone are excellent pure opioid agonists (Table 3).

Mixed opioid agonists provide the benefits of an opioid, while targeting additional pain receptors. Tapentadol, tramadol, duloxetine, and amitriptyline inhibit the reuptake of serotonin and norepinephrine.[36] Caution should be taken to avoid duplicating effects at the same receptor that may increase adverse effects.

Adjuncts for both forms of acute pain consist of regional or local blocks using lidocaine or bupivacaine, NMDA antagonists (ketamine), and antihistamines.[25,26,37] As previously discussed, regional lidocaine and bupivacaine blocks should be considered for procedures and isolated burns to limit systemic drug exposures.[25,26] Ketamine analgesic doses have been shown to reduce postoperative opioid consumption, pain during dressing changes, and the development of burn-related chronic pain.[37] Antihistamines have demonstrated significant improvements in pruritus as early as 1 hour after administration.[38,39] They should be considered for all patients with nociceptive and neuropathic pruritus. Clonidine and dexmedetomidine have demonstrated opioid sparing effects and psychological effects by inhibiting sympathetic outflow signaling of the CNS.[40,41] Epidural, intrathecal and local/topical routes of clonidine may be effective for preventing or managing chronic pain conditions that are primarily neuropathic.[42]

Acute Nociceptive Pain

Acute nociceptive pain base management benefits from acetaminophen/paracetamol, a nonsteroidal anti-inflammatory drug (NSAID), vitamin C, and an opioid or mixed mechanism of action opioid drug. Acetaminophen/paracetamol and NSAIDs are efficacious drugs unique to managing acute nociceptive pain.

Acetaminophen/paracetamol is a weak analgesic that acts both centrally and peripherally to inhibit pain. NSAIDs provide additional benefits of anti-inflammatory effects; however, they may further exacerbate acute kidney injury and should be avoided during the pathophysiologic shock phase. When acetaminophen/paracetamol and NSAIDs were used in multimodal management, synergistic analgesic effects were comparable to a higher opioid dose, with less adverse effects.[43,44]

A muscle relaxant may be used as an adjunct to provide additional short-term benefits for acute nociceptive pain, secondary to muscle overactivity. Muscle overactivity may contribute to nociceptive pain by stimulating the surrounding tissues. Burned patients are often critically ill and immobilized for extended durations in the intensive care unit. During the hypermetabolic burn state, muscle is susceptible to atrophy, spasm, and protein degradation, which can release local and systemic inflammatory markers.

Acute Neuropathic Pain

Acute neuropathic pain base management consists of an antiepileptic (gabapentin or pregabalin), antidepressant (duloxetine), lidocaine, vitamin C, and an opioid or mixed opioid drug. Gabapentin, pregabalin, duloxetine, amitriptyline, and lidocaine are efficacious drugs unique to managing acute neuropathic pain. Gabapentin or pregabalin and duloxetine should be added to base management of all patients with burn-related neuropathic pain.[6,45] These antiepileptics and antidepressants can modulate neurotransmitters and signals, improve healing of axons, fibers, myelin, and prevent the development of chronic pain.[6] If a patient is unable to receive duloxetine, amitriptyline may be used; however, amitriptyline has the disadvantage of a greater number of adverse effects.[46]

Table 3 Equianalgesic opioid conversion table		
Drug	IV/IM (mg)	PO (mg)
Hydrocodone	-	30
Oxycodone	-	20
Hydromorphone	1.5	7.5
Fentanyl	0.1	-

Abbreviations: IM, intramuscular; IV, intravenous; PO, by mouth.

CHRONIC MANAGEMENT

A pharmacologic regimen consisting of a stepwise approach using base management and adjuncts should be tailored to each patient for burn-related chronic neuropathic and/or nociplastic pain (see **Fig. 2**). Lower drug doses should be started and titrated using multimodal targeted management, then titrate doses and add drugs to achieve burn-related pain relief (see **Table 2**). Consider referral to pain management for chronic neuropathic and nociplastic pain states.

Chronic Neuropathic and Nociplastic Pain

Both types of chronic pain may benefit from gabapentin, pregabalin, duloxetine, amitriptyline, and/or vitamin C. Opioids are not preferred for chronic noncancer pain due to insufficient benefits and risks of serious harm. Adjuncts for both forms of chronic pain consist of regional or local blocks using lidocaine or bupivacaine and antihistamines.[25,26,37] Cannabidiol (CBD) has not been approved by the Food and Drug Administration for the management of pain. Randomized controlled trials have consistently demonstrated CBD is no more effective than placebo for neuropathic and nociceptive pain.[47–50]

Chronic Neuropathic Pain

Surgical etiologies of chronic neuropathic pain secondary to direct nerve injury or compression should be considered to avoid long-term unnecessary exposure to pharmacologic agents. If burn-related pain is amenable to surgical interventions, these interventions should be considered.[6,10]

Local or topical lidocaine can attenuate chronic neuropathic pain and reduce pain-related biomedical markers.[51] Lidocaine should be considered for base management of burn-related chronic neuropathic pain. Ketamine may provide similar benefits as an adjunct seen in acute neuropathic pain as chronic neuropathic pain.[37]

Chronic Nociplastic Pain

There are no definitive guidelines for the management of nociplastic pain. This becomes even less clear in the setting of burn-related pain. The pathophysiologic primary and/or secondary sensitization and subsequent neuromodulation in nociplastic pain requires management through mechanisms of relearning. NSAIDs and opioids should be avoided. Elevated concentrations of endogenous opioids can worsen hyperalgesia and alter sleep architecture.[13,14] Low-dose naltrexone, an opioid antagonist, increases the density of opioid receptors, improves the response to endogenous opiates, and improves clinical symptoms.[52,53]

The development and maintenance of pain hypersensitivity has been found to be dependent on the NMDA receptor.[15] Gabapentin binds to presynaptic calcium channels involved in pain hypersensitivity, indirectly inhibits overactivation of the NMDA receptor and limits long-term pain sensitization.[16] Ketamine directly inhibits the NMDA receptor to reduce both primary and secondary hyperalgesia.[18] Methadone, a potent mu-opioid peptide receptor agonist and weak NMDA receptor antagonist, works similarly to reduce OIH.[19]

SUMMARY

- Burn-related pain should be assessed first by chronicity (acute or chronic), followed by type (nociceptive, neuropathic, nociplastic) to guide multimodal pharmacologic management in a stepwise algorithm approach.
- Multimodal pharmacologic management includes knowledge and understanding of pharmacokinetics, pharmacodynamics, pharmacoeconomics, pharmacogenomics, and pharmacotherapeutics.
- Combination therapy increases efficacy and reduces toxicity by offering a multimodal approach to burn-related pain by targeting different receptors in the PNS and CNS.
- Responses to multimodal pharmacologic management should frequently be assessed using the numerical rating scale (NRS) for pain (mild = 1–3; moderate = 4–6; severe = 7–10).
- Consider etiologies of burn-related pain that may be amenable to surgical interventions or chronic pain states that may require a referral to pain management.

CLINICS CARE POINTS

- Set expectations: Set pain expectations at first patient encounter to avoid unrealistic expectations and outcomes.
- Build therapeutic alliance: Build a therapeutic patient alliance through shared decision making to actively involve each patient in their care.
- Prevention: Prevention of chronic pain is the primary goal of acute pain management.
- Identify pain etiologies: Once pain has been established, identify all etiologies of pain as surgical or medical to direct management.
- Individualize management: Pharmacotherapeutic pain management is individualized and likely different for each patient.

DISCLOSURE

This research did not receive any specific grant from funding agencies in the public, commercial, or not-for-profit sectors.

REFERENCES

1. Raja SN, Carr DB, Cohen M, et al. The revised international association for the study of pain definition of pain: concepts, challenges, and compromises. Pain 2020;161(9):1976–82.

2. Morgan M, Deuis JR, Frøsig-Jørgensen M, et al. Burn pain: a systematic and critical review of epidemiology, pathophysiology, and treatment. Pain Med 2018;19(4):708–34.

3. Van Loey NE, Bremer M, Faber AW, et al. Itching following burns: epidemiology and predictors. Br J Dermatol 2008;158(1):95–100.

4. Falch C, Vicente D, Häberle H, et al. Treatment of acute abdominal pain in the emergency room: a systematic review of the literature. Eur J Pain 2014;18(7):902–13.

5. Hjermstad MJ, Fayers PM, Haugen DF, et al. Studies comparing numerical rating scales, verbal rating scales, and visual analogue scales for assessment of pain intensity in adults: a systematic literature review. J Pain Symptom Manag 2011;41(6):1073–93.

6. Klifto KM, Hultman CS, Dellon AL. Nerve pain after burn injury: a proposed etiology-based classification. Plast Reconstr Surg 2021;147(3):635–44.

7. Chung BY, Kim HB, Jung MJ, et al. Post-burn pruritus. Int J Mol Sci 2020;21(11). https://doi.org/10.3390/ijms21113880.

8. Klifto KM, Yesantharao PS, Lifchez SD, et al. Chronic nerve pain after burn injury: an anatomical approach and the development and validation of a model to predict a patient's risk. Plast Reconstr Surg 2021; 148(4):548e–57e.

9. Klifto KM, Dellon AL, Hultman CS. Prevalence and associated predictors for patients developing chronic neuropathic pain following burns. Burns Trauma 2020;8:tkaa011.

10. Klifto KM, Dellon AL, Hultman CS. Risk factors associated with the progression from acute to chronic neuropathic pain after burn-related injuries. Ann Plast Surg 2020;84(6S Suppl 5):S382–5.

11. Klifto KM, Yesantharao PS, Dellon AL, et al. Chronic neuropathic pain following hand burns: etiology, treatment, and long-term outcomes. J Hand Surg Am 2021;46(1):67.e1. https://doi.org/10.1016/j.jhsa.2020.07.001, 67.e9.

12. Sène D, Cacoub P, Authier FJ, et al. Sjögren syndrome-associated small fiber neuropathy: characterization from a prospective series of 40 cases. Medicine (Baltim) 2013;92(5):e10–8.

13. Rosen IM, Aurora RN, Kirsch DB, et al. Chronic opioid therapy and sleep: an American academy of sleep medicine position statement. J Clin Sleep Med 2019;15(11):1671–3.

14. Xia WS, Peng YN, Tang LH, et al. Spinal ephrinB/EphB signalling contributed to remifentanil-induced hyperalgesia via NMDA receptor. Eur J Pain 2014; 18(9):1231–9.

15. Willert RP, Woolf CJ, Hobson AR, et al. The development and maintenance of human visceral pain hypersensitivity is dependent on the N-methyl-D-aspartate receptor. Gastroenterology 2004;126(3): 683–92.

16. Van Elstraete AC, Sitbon P, Mazoit JX, et al. Gabapentin prevents delayed and long-lasting hyperalgesia induced by fentanyl in rats. Anesthesiology 2008;108(3):484–94.

17. Van Elstraete AC, Sitbon P, Benhamou D, et al. The median effective dose of ketamine and gabapentin in opioid-induced hyperalgesia in rats: an isobolographic analysis of their interaction. Anesth Analg 2011;113(3):634–40.

18. Ilkjaer S, Petersen KL, Brennum J, et al. Effect of systemic N-methyl-D-aspartate receptor antagonist (ketamine) on primary and secondary hyperalgesia in humans. Br J Anaesth 1996;76(6):829–34.

19. Axelrod DJ, Reville B. Using methadone to treat opioid-induced hyperalgesia and refractory pain. J Opioid Manag 2007;3(2):113–4.

20. Cuthbertson D. Post-shock metabolic response. Lancet 1942;239(6189):433–7.

21. Blanchet B, Jullien V, Vinsonneau C, et al. Influence of burns on pharmacokinetics and pharmacodynamics of drugs used in the care of burn patients. Clin Pharmacokinet 2008;47(10):635–54.

22. Steele AN, Grimsrud KN, Sen S, et al. Gap analysis of pharmacokinetics and pharmacodynamics in burn patients: a review. J Burn Care Res 2015;36(3):e194–211.

23. Whirl-Carrillo M, Huddart R, Gong L, et al. An evidence-based framework for evaluating pharmacogenomics knowledge for personalized medicine. Clin Pharmacol Ther 2021;110(3):563–72.

24. Wu CL, Cohen SR, Richman JM, et al. Efficacy of postoperative patient-controlled and continuous infusion epidural analgesia versus intravenous patient-controlled analgesia with opioids: a meta-analysis. Anesthesiology 2005;103(5):1079–88. quiz 1109-10.

25. Abdelrahman I, Steinvall I, Elmasry M, et al. Lidocaine infusion has a 25% opioid-sparing effect on background pain after burns: a prospective, randomised, double-blind, controlled trial. Burns 2020; 46(2):465–71.

26. Wasiak J, Spinks A, Costello V, et al. Adjuvant use of intravenous lidocaine for procedural burn pain relief: a randomized double-blind, placebo-controlled, cross-over trial. Burns 2011;37(6):951–7.

27. Keramidas EG, Rodopoulou SG. Ropivacaine versus lidocaine in digital nerve blocks: a prospective study. Plast Reconstr Surg 2007;119(7):2148–52.

28. Cuvillon P, Nouvellon E, Ripart J, et al. A comparison of the pharmacodynamics and pharmacokinetics of bupivacaine, ropivacaine (with epinephrine) and their equal volume mixtures with lidocaine used for femoral and sciatic nerve blocks: a double-blind randomized study. Anesth Analg 2009;108(2):641–9.

29. Dowell D, Ragan KR, Jones CM, et al. Prescribing opioids for pain - the new CDC clinical practice guideline. N Engl J Med 2022;387(22):2011–3.

30. Edwards RR, Dolman AJ, Michna E, et al. Changes in pain sensitivity and pain modulation during oral opioid treatment: the impact of negative affect. Pain Med 2016;17(10):1882–91.

31. Mauermann E, Filitz J, Dolder P, et al. Does fentanyl lead to opioid-induced hyperalgesia in healthy volunteers?: a double-blind, randomized, crossover trial. Anesthesiology 2016;124(2):453–63.

32. Chu LF, Dairmont J, Zamora AK, et al. The endogenous opioid system is not involved in modulation of opioid-induced hyperalgesia. J Pain 2011;12(1):108–15.

33. Afshari R, Maxwell SR, Webb DJ, et al. Morphine is an arteriolar vasodilator in man. Br J Clin Pharmacol 2009;67(4):386–93.

34. Prakash S, Fatima T, Pawar M. Patient-controlled analgesia with fentanyl for burn dressing changes. Anesth Analg 2004;99(2):552–5. table of contents.

35. Linneman PK, Terry BE, Burd RS. The efficacy and safety of fentanyl for the management of severe procedural pain in patients with burn injuries. J Burn Care Rehabil 2000;21(6):519–22.

36. Marks DM, Shah MJ, Patkar AA, et al. Serotonin-norepinephrine reuptake inhibitors for pain control: premise and promise. Curr Neuropharmacol 2009;7(4):331–6.

37. Zor F, Ozturk S, Bilgin F, et al. Pain relief during dressing changes of major adult burns: ideal analgesic combination with ketamine. Burns 2010;36(4):501–5.

38. Baker RA, Zeller RA, Klein RL, et al. Burn wound itch control using H1 and H2 antagonists. J Burn Care Rehabil 2001;22(4):263–8.

39. Ahuja RB, Gupta R, Gupta G, et al. A comparative analysis of cetirizine, gabapentin and their combination in the relief of post-burn pruritus. Burns 2011;37(2):203–7.

40. Viggiano M, Badetti C, Roux F, et al. Analgésie contrôlée par le patient brûlé: effet d'épargne de fentanyl par la clonidine Burn patient controlled analgesia: fentanyl sparing effect of clonidine. Ann Fr Anesth Reanim 1998;17(1):19–26.

41. Kim D, Lee C, Bae H, et al. Comparison of the perfusion index as an index of noxious stimulation in monitored anesthesia care of propofol/remifentanil and propofol/dexmedetomidine: a prospective, randomized, case-control, observational study. BMC Anesthesiol 2023;23(1):183.

42. Kumar A, Maitra S, Khanna P, et al. Clonidine for management of chronic pain: a brief review of the current evidences. Saudi J Anaesth 2014;8(1):92–6.

43. Meyer WJ, Nichols RJ, Cortiella J, et al. Acetaminophen in the management of background pain in children post-burn. J Pain Symptom Manag 1997;13(1):50–5.

44. Pergolizzi JV, Magnusson P, LeQuang JA, et al. Can NSAIDs and acetaminophen effectively replace opioid treatment options for acute pain? Expert Opin Pharmacother 2021;22(9):1119–26.

45. Najafi A, Zeinali Nejad H, Nikvarz N. Evaluation of the analgesic effects of duloxetine in burn patients: an open-label randomized controlled trial. Burns 2019;45(3):598–609.

46. Tesfaye S, Sloan G, Petrie J, et al. Comparison of amitriptyline supplemented with pregabalin, pregabalin supplemented with amitriptyline, and duloxetine supplemented with pregabalin for the treatment of diabetic peripheral neuropathic pain (OPTION-DM): a multicentre, double-blind, randomised crossover trial. Lancet 2022;400(10353):680–90.

47. Arout CA, Haney M, Herrmann ES, et al. A placebo-controlled investigation of the analgesic effects, abuse liability, safety and tolerability of a range of oral cannabidiol doses in healthy humans. Br J Clin Pharmacol 2022;88(1):347–55.

48. De Vita MJ, Maisto SA, Gilmour CE, et al. The effects of cannabidiol and analgesic expectancies on experimental pain reactivity in healthy adults: a balanced placebo design trial. Exp Clin Psychopharmacol 2022;30(5):536–46.

49. Dieterle M, Zurbriggen L, Mauermann E, et al. Pain response to cannabidiol in opioid-induced hyperalgesia, acute nociceptive pain, and allodynia using a model mimicking acute pain in healthy adults in a randomized trial (CANAB II). Pain 2022;163(10):1919–28.

50. Zubcevic K, Petersen M, Bach FW, et al. Oral capsules of tetra-hydro-cannabinol (THC), cannabidiol (CBD) and their combination in peripheral neuropathic pain treatment. Eur J Pain 2023;27(4):492–506.

51. Lin CT, Tsai YJ, Wang HY, et al. Pre-emptive treatment of lidocaine attenuates neuropathic pain and reduces pain-related biochemical markers in the rat cuneate nucleus in median nerve chronic constriction injury model. Anesthesiol Res Pract 2012;2012:921405.

52. King CD, Goodin B, Kindler LL, et al. Reduction of conditioned pain modulation in humans by naltrexone: an exploratory study of the effects of pain catastrophizing. J Behav Med 2013;36(3):315–27.

53. Younger J, Noor N, McCue R, et al. Low-dose naltrexone for the treatment of fibromyalgia: findings of a small, randomized, double-blind, placebo-controlled, counterbalanced, crossover trial assessing daily pain levels. Arthritis Rheum 2013;65(2):529–38.

Update on Cold-Induced Injuries

Francesco M. Egro, MD, MSc, MRCS[a,b,]*, Eva Roy, MD[c,1], Jonathan Friedstat, MD, MPH[d]

KEYWORDS

- Cold-induced injuries • Cold injuries • Frostbite • Frostnip • Thrombolytics • Outcomes

KEY POINTS

- Cold-induced injuries are a major challenge for burn surgeons, leading to significant sequelae for the patients including amputations, long-term disability, and death.
- Rapid assessment and diagnosis are essential for optimal outcomes.
- Various therapies have emerged to improve outcomes. Topical, oral, and intravenous agents have shown to minimize the impact of cold-induced injuries.
- Thrombolytics have shown the greatest promise in improving tissue perfusion outcomes in cold-induced injuries.

INTRODUCTION

Cold-induced injuries (also known as cold injuries or frostbite) are traumatic injuries that occur when a person is exposed to temperatures less than freezing for prolonged periods, leading to direct cellular damage and progressive tissue ischemia. Cold-induced injuries were first brought to light to due to the prevalence in the military. Despite advances in twenty-first century development, cold-induced injuries still occur every day in the urban and rural setting, with unfortunately poor outcomes (**Fig. 1**). This article will discuss the epidemiology, pathophysiology, staging, therapeutics, and outcomes of cold injuries.

EPIDEMIOLOGY

Cold-induced injuries occur when the body is exposed to extreme cold temperatures, leading to tissue damage and adverse health effects. Cold-induced injuries have been prevalent for thousands of years. The oldest known case of frostbite is a mummy found in Chilean mountains from 5000 years ago.[1] Celsus wrote the first description of frostbite.[1] In addition, frostbite became more prevalent with the widespread impact it had on the military. For example, cold-related injuries destroyed majority of Napoleon's army during the invasion of Russia in 1812. Between World War I, World War II, and the Korean War, more than 1 million soldiers were severely affected by cold injuries.[2] In the 2020–2021 winter season, frostbites were the most common type of cold injury among active-duty military, resulting in an incidence of 35.4 per 100,000 person years. A recent study assessing the National Inpatient Sample (2016–2018), demonstrated an overall incidence of cold-induced injuries in the United States of 0.83 of 100,000 people; interestingly, the incidence almost doubled between 2016 (0.66 of 100,000) and 2018 (1.21 of 100,000).[3]

Cold-induced injuries are still prevalent and can affect a wide variety of people from outdoor

[a] Department of Plastic Surgery, University of Pittsburgh Medical Center, 1350 Locust Street, Suite G103, Pittsburgh, PA 15219, USA; [b] Department of Surgery, University of Pittsburgh Medical Center, 1400 Locust Street, Pittsburgh, PA 15219, USA; [c] Division of Plastic Surgery, Massachusetts General Hospital, Harvard Medical School, 55 Fruit Street, Boston, MA 02114, USA; [d] Division of Plastic Surgery, Massachusetts General Hospital, Harvard Medical School, Fraser Outpatient Burn Center, GWB-1300, 55 Fruit Street, Boston, MA 02114, USA
[1] Present address: 4 Emerson Place, Apartment 1007, Boston, MA 02114.
* Corresponding author. Department of Plastic Surgery, University of Pittsburgh Medical Center, 1350 Locus Street, Medical Professional Building, Pittsburgh, PA 15219.
E-mail address: francescoegro@gmail.com

Clin Plastic Surg 51 (2024) 303–311
https://doi.org/10.1016/j.cps.2023.11.005
0094-1298/24/© 2023 Elsevier Inc. All rights reserved.

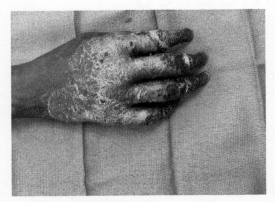

Fig. 1. Right hand fourth-degree cold-induced injury affecting all digits.

workers to hikers at a high altitude to elderly individuals and the homeless population. There are many risk factors for cold injuries. Common behavioral factors that put one at risk for injury is alcohol because it inhibits shivering and causes cutaneous vasodilation that precipitates frostbite at warmer temperatures.[4] Other behavioral factors include drugs such as opioids, marijuana, cocaine, and smoking in addition to access to shelter. Physiologic risk factors include hiking or residing in high altitudes. Comorbidities can also put one at risk for cold-induced injury such as peripheral vascular disease, Raynaud disease, diabetes, neuropathies, and psychiatric illnesses such as schizophrenia. Overall, studies show that cold-induced injuries are more common in men than women with middle-aged men being the most commonly affected.

PATHOPHYSIOLOGY

The skin is the body's largest organ and is responsible for 90% of total heat loss. Hypothermia occurs when core body temperature drops to less than 95°F. Skin can freeze at 28°F, and cold-induced injury occurs when skin is exposed to temperature less than its freezing point.[5]

The body's thermostat is the hypothalamus. As temperature drops, the body responds by increasing heat production and limiting skin blood flow. In addition, peripheral vasoconstriction occurs to preserve temperature and shivering to generate more heat energy. Vasoconstriction helps to conserve heat by reducing blood flow to the skin and extremities, limiting heat loss.

Persistent vasoconstriction and reduced blood leads to tissue ischemia. Ischemia leads to impaired cellular metabolism and function with a decrease in oxygen and nutrient delivery to the tissues. As tissues cool, extracellular fluid in the

tissues may freeze forming ice crystals. Ice crystal formation can lead to mechanical damage to cells and disrupt cellular structures.

At the cellular level, ice crystal formation and ischemia result in cellular injury. Ice crystals cause mechanical damage to cell membrane and organelles, denaturation of lipid–protein complexes, and thermal shock.[5] The combination of reduced blood flow, ischemia, and direct cellular injury leads to cellular dysfunction and eventual cell death.

Subsequently, an inflammatory response occurs. Once rewarming begins, reperfusion injury can occur. During reperfusion, the sudden restoration of blood flow to previously ischemic tissues can lead to the release of reactive oxygen species and formation of free radicals. Reperfusion injury exacerbated tissue damage by inducing oxidative stress, inflammation, and additional cellular injury. In addition to reperfusion injury, progressive microvascular insult due to microvascular thrombosis can occur resulting in continued cell injury. This secondary response including increased inflammatory mediators, free radicals, thrombosis, and reperfusion injury contribute to progressive dermal ischemia.[6]

CLASSIFICATION OF COLD-INDUCED INJURIES

Multiple ways exist to classify and stage cold-induced injuries. Frostbite progresses from superficial to deep. The initial stage is frostnip, which is the superficial form of local freezing. Symptoms include anesthesia, paresthesia, and a white or pale appearance of skin. This form is mild and is completely reversible. There is no ice crystal formation or microvascular injury and importantly no tissue loss. On rewarming, the skin becomes red and may be accompanied by some swelling or pain but there is no long-term tissue damage. This is most commonly seen on the hands and face.

Frostnip then progresses to superficial frostbite, which is when the top layers of the skin freeze. Symptoms include skin that is pale, hard, cold, anesthesia, erythema, and skin vesicles. The tissue freezes slowly and forms ice crystals. There can be clear or milky fluid present within the blisters and surrounding edema. On rewarming, skin may seem mottled, bluish, or reddish purple.

The final stage is deep frostbite, which occurs when the deeper layers of the skin as well as the tissues beneath are affected. Symptoms include development of hard, cold, and pale skin that has a waxy appearance. Individuals may experience complete anesthesia, and joint stiffness. Blisters and hemorrhagic blisters may form indicating injury into reticular dermis and beneath the dermal vascular plexus.[7] The tissue necrosis can extend to muscle or bone. Severe cases may result in tissue death and gangrene. See **Table 1** for summary of classification.

There is also a staging classification similar to the burn classification system based on degrees.[7] First degree is superficial injury with reduced sensation, central pallor, and surrounding erythema. With first degree, there are no long-term consequences. Second-degree injury occurs within the dermis and includes skin blistering with surrounding erythema, edema. Third-degree injury includes tissue involving entire thickness of skin and can lead to hemorrhagic blisters. Fourth-degree injury is when tissue loss involves deeper structures beneath the skin such as muscle tendon and bone resulting in mottled cyanotic skin (**Fig. 2**).

There is also a grading classification based on cold injury effecting upper and lower extremities developed by Cauchy and colleagues.[8] Grade 1 is when there is no cyanosis on the extremity and no risk of amputation. Grade 2 is cyanosis on distal phalanx only, amputation to soft tissue and sequelae of fingernail/toenail predicted. Grade 3 is cyanosis on intermediate and proximal phalanx. Amputation to the bone of the digit and functional sequelae predicted. Grade 4 is cyanosis over carpal and tarsal bones, amputation to limb and functional sequelae predicted. The increase in grade leads to increase in likelihood of limb amputation.

INITIAL MANAGEMENT OF COLD-INDUCED INJURIES

The initial treatment protocol developed by Robson and Heggers at University of Chicago in 1983 is still the basis for treatment guidelines today.[9] This consists of rapid rewarming, pain control, tetanus prophylaxis, and limb elevation.

The rewarming process is usually best accomplished in a medical facility. However, the decision of whether to start the rewarming process in the field is based on whether the transport time outside of the cold environment to a medical facility is less than 2 hours. If the expected transport time is greater than 2 hours, then the priority should be to prevent or treat hypothermia. Tissues that are thawed and then refrozen will become severely injured and will likely be lost. Cold-induced injuries should be handled with care to avoid further trauma. All constricting clothing or jewelry should be removed. Smoking or use of nicotine products should be avoided to minimize peripheral vascular compromise.

The rewarming process is recommended by the from the State of Alaska Department of Health and Social Services state to be performed using a warm water bath a temperature of 37°C to 39°C (99°F–102°F) for 20 to 45 minutes or until tissues become flushed, soft, and pliable.[10] The water should be circulated to maintain a consistent temperature and prevent burns. Rewarming can be extremely painful, and administration of analgesia should be considered. Nonsteroidal anti-inflammatory drugs (NSAIDs) or opioids can be used; NSAIDs are usually a first-line choice for its dual pain control and anti-inflammatory effect. Cold-induced injuries are prone to tetanus; therefore, tetanus immunization should be verified and updated as needed. The use of prophylactic systemic antibiotic is controversial. Older studies seem to recommend its use to prevent a superimposed infection in patients with severe edema because of loss of the protective properties of the skin against skin flora.[11] However, more recent recommendations from the State of Alaska Department of Health and Social Services state that antibiotics are not necessary except for prophylaxis of grossly contaminated wounds or treatment of established infection. Recent studies have shown that the microflora of cold-injuries wounds

Table 1
Classification of frostbites

Classification	Tissue Affected	Symptoms/Signs	Outcomes
Frostnip	Epidermis	Anesthesia, paresthesia, and skin pallor	Reversible
Superficial frostbite	Epidermis and superficial dermis	Skin pallor, firmness, anesthesia, erythema, and edema clear blisters	Good outcomes
Deep frostbite	Deep dermis, fat, muscle, tendon, and bone	Skin pallor, firmness, anesthesia, waxy appearance, joint stiffness, blisters ± hemorrhagic blisters, and gangrene	Poor outcomes

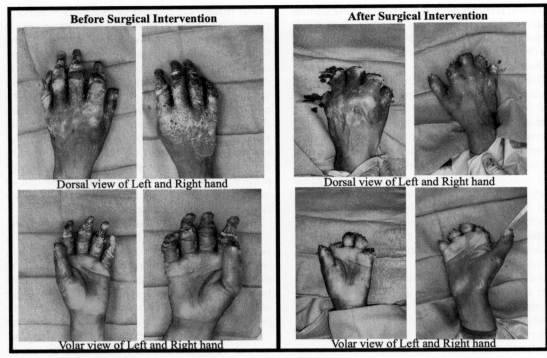

Before Surgical Intervention

Dorsal view of Left and Right hand

Volar view of Left and Right hand

After Surgical Intervention

Dorsal view of Left and Right hand

Volar view of Left and Right hand

Fig. 2. Representative case of bilateral hand fourth-degree frostbites requiring 10-digit amputation.

include a mixture of gram-negative and gram-positive bacteria.[9,12] *Pseudomonas aeruginosa* seems to be the most common among gram-negative bacteria (17.9%), whereas *Staphylococcus aureus* was the most common among gram-positive bacteria (21.1%). The authors also showed the high resistance of these bacteria to ciprofloxacin (66.6%), erythromycin (52.5%), and lincomycin (44.4%).

After rewarming, blisters may form. Small blisters may be left intact but large blisters may need to be unroofed especially if they are causing functional impairment. If warranted, blisters can be unroofed at bedside and open wounds should be cleaned, dressed with sterile dressing, protected from further injury, splinted, and elevated. A concern exists about unroofing hemorrhagic blisters because they are likely a sequela of damage of deeper structures. Robsons and Heggers examined blister fluid in early phase frostbite wounds and found that the vasoconstricting metabolites of arachidonic acid, PgF2 alpha and TxB2, were elevated.[13] These are known to be involved in dermal ischemia in burns and pedicle flaps, and thus are likely to play a role in the pathogenesis of cold-induced injuries. Therefore, many therapies have aimed to counteract the arachidonic acid cascade and minimize dermal ischemia. Various topical, oral, and intravenous

agents have been used including topical antimicrobials, methimazole, aloe vera, aspirin, ibuprofen, methylprednisolone, pentoxifylline, iloprost, and thrombolytics.

Heggers and colleagues[14] showed that tissue survival was improved with methimazole (34.3%), aloe vera (28.2%), aspirin (22.5%), and methylprednisolone (17.5%). Miller and Koltai showed that the addition of pentoxifylline to aloe vera improved tissue survival even further (30%) when compared with control (6%), pentoxifylline alone (20%), and aloe vera cream alone (24%).[15]

Aloe vera is a potent antiprostaglandin agent that inhibits the arachidonic acid pathway and, thus, might decrease the detrimental effects of the prostaglandin cascade in cold-tissue injuries.[16,17] Nonsteroidal anti-inflammatories also reduce prostaglandin activity, thus reducing the inflammatory damage. Aspirin was historically recommended due to its inhibitory effect of the arachidonic acid pathway; however, it also blocks metabolites that are beneficial for wound healing. For this reason, some authors advocate for the use of ibuprofen (600–800 mg every 6 hours) instead to specifically target TXA_2 blockade.[11] Pentoxifylline is a phosphodiesterase inhibitor that has shown to decrease blood viscosity, increase red blood cell flexibility, decreases platelet hyperactivity, helps normalize the prostacyclin-tothromboxane A2 ratio, and increases perfusion to the affected extremity.[18] Studies have used it in pedal frostbites prescribed as 400 mg 3 times a day for 2 to 6 weeks. Iloprost is a synthetic prostacyclin analog that leads to vasodilation, inhibition of platelet aggregation, and cytoprotection.[19] Intravenous administration of iloprost has been shown to be effective in reducing amputations up to 48 hours after rewarming.[20,21]

Thrombolytics have shown the greatest promise in improving tissue perfusion outcomes in cold-induced injuries. The most commonly used agent is tissue plasminogen activator (t-PA), which activates plasminogen, which yields the proteolytic enzyme plasmin, which in turn breaks the links between fibrin molecules. This disrupts the integrity of blood clots and restores blood flow.[16] It can be administered intravenously or intra-arterially,[22] and no studies exist comparing the impact of intravenous and intra-arterial thrombolytic administration on amputation rate or on the impact of level of amputation. Bruen and colleagues[23] showed that patients who received t-PA within 24 hours of injury had improved tissue perfusion and decreased rates of amputations compared with patients who did not. The incidence of digital amputation in patients who did not receive t-PA was 41% versus 10% in those patients who did receive t-PA within 24 hours of injury.[23] Carmichael and colleagues[24] conducted a retrospective review with a larger cohort of patients showed increased limb salvage rates with administration of t-PA. They also examined the benefit of prehospital administration of t-PA and found significant risk reduction in amputation for patients who received t-PA at an outside center.[24] The only prospective trial was described by Cauchy and colleagues,[20] where they demonstrated iloprost in addition to IV t-PA decreased amputations compared with control group (19% vs 60%, $P = .03$). Intravenous t-PA is now considered a part of routine protocol when there are absent Doppler signals after rewarming or limited perfusion shown by bone scans because it decreases rates of amputations.[25,26] Contraindications to thrombolytic therapy include significant concurrent trauma, pregnancy, recent surgery or hemorrhage within 10 days, or intracranial bleeding within 3 months. Relative contraindications to thrombolytic therapy include moderate concurrent trauma, prolonged warm ischemia time, and multiple freeze–thaw cycles.[27] A limitation in the use of thrombolytics is the concern for bleeding complications.

Intra-arterial t-PA has also been used when there is no improvement on rapid rewarming, absent Doppler pulses, limited perfusion on bone scan. Catheter-directed thrombolytics therapy may be more effective than systemic therapy.[28] Patel and colleagues[29] demonstrated that intra-arterial thrombolysis reduced digital amputation rates and hospital length of stay. These patients require IV heparin, daily aspirin, continuous monitoring of fibrinogen level, partial thromboplastin time, and complete blood count.

Some potential adjunctive treatments include hyperbaric oxygen (HBO). This was first described by Leginham in 1963.[30] Various case reports have shown that it can help to increase oxygen delivery, decrease edema, promote bacteriologic control, and increase erythrocyte flexibility.[31–33] Ghumman and colleagues[34] showed in their retrospective cohort study of 22 patients treated with anticoagulation and HBO that all recovered without soft tissue damage or amputations. Of note 72.7% of patients did experience at least 1 side effect of HBO, including nausea, vomiting, anxiety, otologic barotrauma, oxygen toxicity seizure, and myopic changes. A study by Magnan and colleagues[35] has shown that the combination of HBO and iloprost compared with iloprost alone, was associated with higher benefit in patients with severe frostbite including a reduction of amputations. HBO does not remain a part of routine protocol because there is no clear evidence for its benefit and should be considered on a case-by-case basis.

Theis and colleagues[36] have described anticoagulation therapy for acute treatment of frostbite as an effective adjunct in reducing amputation and length of stay. However, anticoagulation after treatment of frostbite remains controversial.[37] There are limited data to support the use of anticoagulation therapy after being discharged. There are also risks of discharging patients on anticoagulation. Currently, the ABA does not have guidelines to support the use of anticoagulation in standard protocol. Sheridian and colleagues[7] includes 72 hours of postlysis heparinization if thrombolytics have been administered and a prophylactic dose of low molecular weight heparin if it has not. Outpatient anticoagulant is best decided on a case-by-case basis.

Sympathetic nerve blocks have also been explored as a means to provide analgesia and therapeutic benefits. Various blocks have been used with mixed outcomes. Syposs and colleagues used a permanent axillary plexus block for the treatment of cold-induced injuries of the upper extremities.[38] However, amputation had to be performed in 20% of cases. Prolonged epidural anesthesia with lidocaine in 91 lower extremity cold-injuries led to an improvement in clinical course and reduction in hospital stay with no amputations.[39] More recently, Chandran and colleagues[40] showed that a distal volar forearm block (10 cc of 1% lidocaine with 1:100,000 epinephrine) leads to warmer finger temperature for during the first 2 hours after the nerve block because of vasodilatation in most patients. Calder and colleagues[41] subsequently showed that bupivacaine digital blocks (with and without epinephrine) lead to pain relief and fingertip hyperemia with consistent fingertip temperature elevation that lasts 15 hours. Although small and preliminary studies, further research is needed to explore the true benefits of sympathetic blockade.

IMAGING

Imaging can be a useful tool in adjunct to physical examination to determine the viability of tissue. Digital subtraction angiography is useful to evaluate perfusion and can help identify targets for therapeutic intervention.[42] Multiphase bone scintigraphy with hybrid single photon emission computed tomography (SPECT)/computed tomography (CT) has shown to be increasingly useful after the initial treatment to determine what tissue is viable. Triple phase bone scans using technetium 99 m pertechnetate have shown utility in determining blood flow. In 1989, Mehta and Wilson recommend obtaining bone scans 48 hours after admission.[43] They found 3 patterns of imaging. The first pattern showed hyperemic flow with an increased blood-pool phase and normal delayed scans of the skeleton and soft tissues; this pattern indicates mild ischemia that required observation and no intervention. The second pattern showed absent blood flow, with no blood-pool images but normal depiction of bone uptake in delayed scans; this pattern indicates ischemia with occasional superficial tissue infarction that required minor debridement. The third pattern showed absent blood pool with absent bone uptake in delayed images; this pattern indicates deep tissue and bone infarction that requires amputation. The combination of SPECT/CT with multiphase bone scintigraphy allows for precise localization of tissue necrosis even before it appears on physical examination. Therefore, multiphase bone scintigraphy with SPECT/CT is increasingly becoming the modality of choice.[9] Finally, MRI/MRA can also be used to evaluate perfusion in digits and extremities and can provide more accurate mapping of the vessels allowing for a clearer line between viable and nonviable tissue. There does not seem to be sufficient evidence supporting the theory that imaging affects the use or the time of initiation of thrombolytic therapy.[27]

OPERATIVE INTERVENTION

Surgery is rarely indicated in the acute setting. Typically, operative intervention is not needed because bedside debridement can be done for superficial blisters. Local wound care is done initially. Of note, compartment syndrome may develop after rewarming of the extremities, potentially requiring fasciotomies. Surgery may be needed after the initial presentation for debridement after clinical demarcation has occurred, typically 2 to 4 weeks after rewarming. This may require debridement and possible digit/limb amputation. During this period, it is important to maintain adequate nutrition to promote optimal wound healing; patients should be encouraged to follow a high protein and high calorie diet.

OUTCOMES

Cold injuries can have long-term consequences that may persist after the initial incident and treatment. In severe cases of frostbite, where tissue necrosis leads to gangrene, surgical amputation may be the only option. Sensory and motor dysfunction may also occur leading to cold sensitivity, sensory loss, decreased sensation, and altered temperature perception. Motor dysfunction including muscle weakness and reduced range of motion may occur. There can also be musculoskeletal-related consequences including localized osteopenia, subchondral bone loss, and joint contractures. Chronic pain including neuropathic pain may occur. This pain is typically characterized by tingling, burning, or shooting sensations. Finally, cold injuries can have an emotional and psychological impact. Amputations and disfigurement can lead to emotional distress, depression, anxiety, and body image issues.

According to the Centers for Disease Control and Prevention, there are approximately 1301 deaths each year in the United States attributed to cold-related injury.[44] In addition to fatalities, there are many nonfatal cold injuries that occur each year such as frostbite and trench foot.

National studies report an amputation rate in severe cold-induced injuries to be between 20% and 30%.[44] Interestingly, studies have shown that the primary amputation revision rate was required in 24% of cases,[45] whereas patients with moderate finger frostbite injuries have developed several sequelae including hypersensitivity to cold (53%), digit anesthesia (40%), or not being able to work at the same level before injury (13%).[46] Another study looking at of US military cold-injuries showed that 67% of patients reported persistent symptoms of neurovascular injury 6 months following frostbite injury and 8% had to be reassigned due to injury.[47] This is evidence that cold-induced injuries lead to long-term disability and sequelae. For these reasons, patients need to be counseled and followed up appropriately.

Frostbite injuries are also a significant burden on hospital resources. Nygaard and Endorf showed that frostbite injuries led to a significantly higher cost and utilization of resources compared with similarly nonfrostbite injuries.[48,49] Furthermore, unplanned readmission rate following cold-induced injuries was very high with a total cost of US$236,872 and a length of hospital stay of 34.7 days.[48]

Outcomes may be improved by early referral and transportation of severe frostbite injuries to burn centers in order to screen for eligibility for thrombolytics and expedite definitive treatment. Potential barriers to treatment and improvement of outcomes in this population include knowledge gaps, prompt identification of severity, timely referral to burn centers, delays in patients seeking care, and contraindications to thrombolytics therapy. The American Burn Association recommends including updated frostbite management in the Advanced Burn Life Support and Advanced Trauma Life Support courses.[27]

SUMMARY

Cold-induced injuries are a major challenge for burn surgeons, leading to significant sequelae for the patients including amputations, long-term disability, and death. Despite the beneficial impact of thrombolytics on outcomes, frostbites remain a significant burden on hospital resources. A paucity of evidence exists preventing the burn surgery community to come to definitive conclusions on key questions and an optimal protocol to manage cold-induced injuries. Future research is needed to understand.

CLINICS CARE POINTS

- Rapid assessment and diagnosis are important to reduce morbidity and optimize outcomes.
- Thrombolytics asdministered within 24 hours have shown the greatest promise in improving tissue perfusion outcomes in cold-inudced injuries.
- Other topical, orla and intravenous therapies should be considered as adjuncts.
- Imaging can be a useful tool in adjunct to physical examination to determine the viability of tissue.
- Surgery is rarely indicated, requiring debridement and possible digit/limb amputation.

CONFLICT OF INTEREST

The authors declare no conflict of interest.

DISCLOSURE

Financial disclosure: the authors have nothing to disclose.

REFERENCES

1. Post PW, Donner DD. Frostbite in a pre-Columbian mummy. Am J Phys Anthropol 1972;37:187–91.
2. Shenaq DS, Gottlieb LJ. Cold injuries. Hand Clin 2017;33(2):257–67.
3. Endorf FW, Nygaard RM. Social determinants of poor outcomes following frostbite injury: a study of the national inpatient sample. J Burn Care Res 2021;42:1261–5.
4. Endorf FW, Nygaard RM. Socioeconomic and co-morbid factors associated with frostbite injury in the United States. J Burn Care Res 2022;43(3):646–51.
5. Handford C, Thomas O, Imray CHE. Frostbite. Emerg Med Clin North Am 2017;35(2):281–99.
6. Mohr WJ, Jenabzadeh K, Ahrenholz DH. Cold injury. Hand Clin 2009;25(4):481–96.
7. Sheridan RL, Goverman JM, Walker TG. Diagnosis and treatment of frostbite. N Engl J Med 2022;386(23):2213–20.
8. Cauchy E, Chetaille E, Marchand V, et al. Retrospective study of 70 cases of severe frostbite lesions: a proposed new classification scheme. Wilderness Environ Med 2001;12(4):248–55.
9. McCauley RL, Hing DN, Robson MC, et al. Frostbite injuries: a rational approach based on the pathophysiology. J Trauma 1983;23(2):143–7.
10. Zafren K, Giesbrecht G. State of Alaska cold injuries guidelines. Juneau (AK): Department of Health and Social Services of Alaska; 2014. p. 29–34.
11. Petrone P, Kuncir EJ, Asensio JA. Surgical management and strategies in the treatment of hypothermia and cold injury. Emerg Med Clin North Am 2003;21(4):1165–78.
12. Shakirov BM. Frostbite in hot climates of Central Asia: retrospective analysis of the microflora of wound and antibiotic therapy. Int J Burns Trauma 2022;12(3):93–7.
13. Robson MC, Heggers JP. Evaluation of hand frostbite blister fluid as a clue to pathogenesis. J Hand Surg Am 1981;6(1):43–7.
14. Heggers JP, Robson MC, Manavalen K, et al. Experimental and clinical observations on frostbite. Ann Emerg Med 1987;16(9):1056–62.
15. Miller MB, Koltai PJ. Treatment of experimental frostbite with pentoxifylline and aloe vera cream. Arch Otolaryngol Head Neck Surg 1995;121(6):678–80.

16. Handford C, Buxton P, Russell K, et al. Frostbite: a practical approach to hospital management. Extrem Physiol Med 2014;3:7.

17. Imray C, Grieve A, Dhillon S, Caudwell Xtreme Everest Research Group. Cold damage to the extremities: frostbite and non-freezing cold injuries. Postgrad Med J 2009;85(1007):481–8.

18. Hayes DW Jr, Mandracchia VJ, Considine C, et al. Pentoxifylline. Adjunctive therapy in the treatment of pedal frostbite. Clin Pod Med Surg 2000;17(4): 715–22.

19. Grant SM, Goa KL. Iloprost. A review of its pharmacodynamic and pharmacokinetic properties, and therapeutic potential in peripheral vascular disease, myocardial ischaemia and extracorporeal circulation procedures. Drugs 1992;43(6):889–924.

20. Cauchy E, Cheguillaume B, Chetaille E. A controlled trial of a prostacyclin and rt-PA in the treatment of severe frostbite. N Engl J Med 2011;364:189–90.

21. Groechenig E. Treatment of frostbite with iloprost. Lancet 1994;344(8930):1152–3.

22. Jenabzadeh K, Mohr WJ, Ahernholz DH. Frostbite: a single institution's twenty year experience with intraarterial thrombolytic therapy [abstract]. J Burn Care Res 2009;30:S103.

23. Bruen KJ, Ballard JR, Morris SE, et al. Reduction of the incidence of amputation in frostbite injury with thrombolytic therapy. Arch Surg 2007;142(6): 546–53.

24. Carmichael H, Michel S, Smith TM, et al. Remote delivery of thrombolytics prior to transfer to a regional burn center for tissue salvage in frostbite: a single-center experi- ence of 199 patients. J Burn Care Res 2022;43:54–60.

25. Johnson AR, Jensen HL, Peltier G, et al. Efficacy of intravenous tissue plasminogen activator in frostbite patients and presentation of a treatment protocol for frostbite patients. Foot Ankle Spec 2011; 4(6):344–8.

26. Gonzaga T, Jenabzadeh K, Anderson CP, et al. Use of intra-arterial thrombolytic therapy for acute treatment of frostbite in 62 patients with review of thrombolytic therapy in frostbite. J Burn Care Res 2016; 37(4):e323–34.

27. Wibbenmeyer L, Lacey AM, Endorf FW, et al. American burn association clinical practice guidelines on the treatment of severe frostbite. J Burn Care Res 2023. https://doi.org/10.1093/jbcr/irad022. irad022.

28. Tavri S, Ganguli S, Bryan RG Jr, et al. Catheter-directed intraarterial thrombolysis as part of a multidisciplinary management protocol of frostbite injury. J Vasc Interv Radiol 2016;27(8):1228–35.

29. Patel N, Srinivasa DR, Srinivasa RN, et al. Intra-arterial thrombolysis for extremity frostbite decreases digital amputation rates and hospital length of stay. Cardiovasc Intervent Radiol 2017;40(12): 1824–31.

30. Ledingham IM, Norman JN, Karasewich. Treatment of clostridial infection with hyperbaric oxygen drenaching. Lancet 1963;1(7277):384.

31. Ward MP, Garnham JR, Simpson BR, et al. Frostbite: general observations and report of cases treated by hyperbaric oxygen. Proc R Soc Med 1968;61(8):787–9.

32. von Heimburg D, Noah EM, Sieckmann UP, et al. Hyperbaric oxygen treatment in deep frostbite of both hands in a boy. Burns 2001;27(4):404–8.

33. Finderle Z, Cankar K. Delayed treatment of frostbite injury with hyperbaric oxygen therapy: a case report. Aviat Sp Env Med 2002;73(4):392–4.

34. Ghumman A, St Denis-Katz H, Ashton R, et al. Treatment of frostbite with hyperbaric oxygen therapy: a single center's experience of 22 cases. Wounds 2019;31(12):322–5.

35. Magnan DM, Gelsomino M, Louge P, et al. Successful delayed hyperbaric oxygen therapy and iloprost treatment on severe frostbite at high altitude. High Alt Med Biol 2022;23(3):294–7.

36. Theis FV, O'Connor WR, Wahl FJ. Anticoagulants in acute frostbite. J Am Med Assoc 1951;146(11): 992–5.

37. Zaramo TZ, Green JK, Janis JE. Practical review of the current management of frostbite injuries. Plast Reconstr Surg Glob Open 2022;10(10):e4618.

38. Syposs T, Novák J, Barna B, et al. Treatment of frostbites of the upper extremities with prolonged blockade of axillary plexus. Acta Chir Plast 1989; 31(3):163–71.

39. Loskutnikov AF, Myshkov GA. Prolongirovannaia épidural'naia anesteziia pri lechenii obmorozheniĭ [Prolonged epidural anesthesia in the treatment of frostbite]. Khirurgiia 2000;(3):42–3.

40. Chandran GJ, Chung B, Lalonde J, et al. The hyperthermic effect of a distal volar forearm nerve block: a possible treatment of acute digital frostbite injuries? Plast Reconstr Surg 2010;126(3):946–50.

41. Calder K, Chung B, O'Brien C, et al. Bupivacaine digital blocks: how long is the pain relief and temperature elevation? Plast Reconstr Surg 2013;131(5): 1098–104.

42. Millet JD, Brown RK, Levi B, et al. Frostbite: spectrum of imaging findings and guidelines for management. Radiographics 2016;36(7):2154–69.

43. Mehta RC, Wilson MA. Frostbite injury: prediction of tissue viability with triple-phase bone scanning. Radiology 1989;170(2):511–4.

44. QuickStats: Number of hypothermia-related deaths,* by sex — national vital statistics system, United States,1999–2011. 2013. Available at: https://www.cdc.gov/mmwr/preview/mmwrhtml/mm6151a6.htm.

45. Endorf FW, Nygaard RM. High cost and resource utilization of frost- bite readmissions in the United States. J Burn Care Res 2021;42:857–64.

46. Coward A, Endorf FW, Nygaard RM. Revision surgery following severe frostbite injury compared to

similar hand and foot burns. J Burn Care Res 2022; 43(5):1015–8.

47. Ervasti O, Hassi J, Rintamäki H, et al. Sequelae of moderate finger frostbite as assessed by subjective sensations, clinical signs, and thermophysiological responses. Int J Circumpolar Health 2000;59:137–45.

48. Taylor MS, Kulungowski MA, Hamelink JK. Frostbite injuries during winter maneuvers: a long-term disability. Mil Med 1989;154(8):411–2.

49. Nygaard RM, Endorf FW. Frostbite vs burns: increased cost of care and Use of hospital resources. J Burn Care Res 2018;39(5):676–9.

Burns in the Elderly

Lux Shah, MD, MPH[a], Audra T. Clark, MD[b],*, Jessica Ballou, MD[c]

KEYWORDS

- Burn injury • Elderly • Aging

KEY POINTS

- Older adults are a growing segment within the global population and are vulnerable to burn injuries.
- Pre-injury comorbidities and frailty may be better predictors of outcomes than chronologic age.
- The exposure to fire risks, including those related to older homes, appliances, or home oxygen, is a significant source of burn injury in the elderly.
- Physiologic changes associated with aging predispose older persons to slower wound healing, but reconstructive options ranging from skin substitutes to grafts and flaps may be suited for elderly burn patients.
- Shared decision-making with patients and caregivers is essential for determining goal-oriented treatment plans.

INTRODUCTION

According to the World Health Organization, by 2030, one in six persons globally will be over the age of 60 years.[1] In the 2020 census, one in six persons in the United States was over the age of 65 years, with the expectation that there will be one in five by 2040. Further, the US Bureau of Labor Statistics estimates that people aged 75 years or older will be the only age group whose labor force participation is projected to increase from 8.9% in 2020 to 11.7% by 2030.[2] With a growing number of older adults within the overall population and the workforce, an increase is expected in elderly burn patients who will need treatment within the community or at designated burn centers.

Considerable progress has been made in burn care resulting in improved outcomes—except in the elderly. The lethal dose 50% in burn patients aged 65 years or older within the United States has remained stable at around 30% to 35% of total body surface area (TBSA).[3]

Defining Elderly: Age Versus Frailty

The definition of "elderly" is heavily debated within the literature, as chronologic age may not reflect physiologic age or frailty. Historically, reaching the age 65 years, or the age of retirement, has signified being elderly. Newer evaluations, however, reserve the term "elderly" for advanced ages (70, 75, or even 80 years or older), reflecting the collective understanding that health interventions, genetics, environment, and resources can result in various health conditions at any age.[4]

There are many different frailty scores, but the Canadian Study of Health and Aging Clinical Frailty Scale and its more recent version—the Clinical Frailty Scale—are most cited in burn literature.[4] Generally, higher age and comorbidities suggest higher frailty. In a large 2020 study that examined frailty during admission in burn patients, higher frailty scores were strongly associated with higher TBSA percentage injuries, longer intensive care unit stays, higher cost per day, and higher 30-day mortality. Many researchers and institutions are shifting away from "elderly" being age-defined but instead favor frailty to better describe an individual's physiologic reserve. Frailty refers to poor pre-injury health and includes factors such as fitness, comorbidities, and dependence, although no internationally recognized standard definition exists. Several frailty score studies

[a] UT Southwestern Department of Surgery, University of Texas Southwestern Medical Center, Dallas, TX, USA; [b] UT Southwestern Division of Burn, Trauma, Acute and Critical Care Surgery, UT Southwestern Medical Center, 5323 Harry Hines Boulevard, Dallas, TX 75390-9159, USA; [c] Johns Hopkins Department of Plastic and Reconstructive Surgery, Johns Hopkins Burn Center, 4940 Eastern Avenue, Baltimore, MD 21224, USA
* Corresponding author.
E-mail address: Audra.Clark@UTSouthwestern.edu

Clin Plastic Surg 51 (2024) 313–318
https://doi.org/10.1016/j.cps.2023.11.006
0094-1298/24/Published by Elsevier Inc.

demonstrate that frail individuals have worse outcomes for many conditions, including burns.[5–9]

For this article's purpose, the authors use the more prevalent definition of "elderly" within the literature as referring to an age greater than 65 years with the understanding that frailty and ability to tolerate injury and recovery may play the predominant role in outcomes.

Physiologic Changes in the Elderly

Aging is associated with physiologic changes that place older adults at higher risk of injury and for difficulty with recovery. Elderly persons typically have diminished alertness, slower reaction times, and decreased mobility.[10] This lack of awareness can exacerbate potential threats, such as a reduced ability to smell mercaptan in a gas leak or the inability to move away from an active fire that could lead to worse inhalation or flame injuries. Aging is also associated with decreased thermal perception stemming from physiologic neuropathy due to decreased cutaneous thermoreceptor density and reduced superficial skin blood flow. Diabetes, which affects approximately 20% of elderly persons in the United States, exacerbates this effect.[11] Decreased sensation within extremities and reduced mobility can make an individual more prone to scald or flame burn. Decreased blood flow and chronic inflammatory states, commonly found in the elderly, also lead to immunosenescence and reduced wound healing.[12]

The physiologic changes of aging also make recovery after a burn more difficult. Aging leads to a thinning of the skin, which means that a burn injury that might only be partial thickness in a younger person will often be full thickness in an elderly patient. Aged skin also shows decreased angiogenesis, impaired lymphatic drainage, and increased edema. Undernutrition and protein malnutrition are also much more common in older patients, further impairing wound healing.

ELDERLY SPECIFIC BURN INJURIES
Household Hazards

The most common burn injuries in older people are flame or scald burns within a household setting.[13] Ever-changing technologies and safety standards have addressed or replaced previously identified burn hazards. Elderly persons, however, tend to own older appliances disproportionately or reside in homes subject to older building codes. Hazardous devices that can produce a flame burn include open flame gas stoves, space heaters with exposed hot coils, and open fireplaces. A 2020 study examined the products implicated in burn injuries in the elderly and found that hot water, open flames, and clothing are the largest sources of burn injuries.[14]

Home Oxygen and the Risk of Injury

Patients on home oxygen therapy who continue to smoke are at significant risk for burn injury.[15] One study found that the burn injury hazard ratio in patients with chronic obstructive pulmonary disease who had been prescribed oxygen was 1.68 (95% CI 1.42–2.00), with an increased hazard ratio among those with lower socioeconomic status.[16] In 2022, the American Burn Association released a position statement on home oxygen burn prevention. Specifically, it cited patient education, smoking cessation therapies, enhancements to equipment safety by medical suppliers (including thermal fuses), and clinician risk assessments when prescribing home oxygen as key to minimizing or preventing home oxygen-associated burns.[17]

MANAGEMENT OF ACUTE BURNS IN THE ELDERLY
Resuscitation in the Elderly

Inflammatory and metabolic responses to stress differ between elderly burn patients and their adult counterparts, often making resuscitation more difficult. Significant burns (> 20% TBSA) require large volumes of crystalloid fluid resuscitation to maintain perfusion, but this can be particularly challenging in patients with poor cardiac or renal function. Elderly burn patients have decreased cardiac efficiency, which is associated with increased preload and resistance, leading to reduced output, hypoperfusion, and sometimes organ failure. Indeed, patients with heart failure are particularly susceptible to fluid overload. High fluid accumulation values are significantly associated with higher in-hospital mortality.[18] As a result, many techniques have been suggested to manage fluids safely. Although the simplest method is to follow a standard "one size fits all" formula such as the Parkland formula and Brooke formula, newer methods include following physiologic endpoints such as urine output or respiratory variation of the inferior vena cava, allowing for more individualized resuscitation[19] Fluid resuscitation should be a dynamic process directed by patient response with the goal of adequate end-organ perfusion with the smallest volume of fluid given. Computer-assisted technologies, such as the Burn Navigator, can aid resuscitation by accounting for several factors, including TBSA percentage burned, age, weight, and urine output.[20] Although such technologies allow for a more tailored fluid regimen for patients, none of these methods specifically account for the limitations that preexisting conditions such as heart failure or renal insufficiency may have on fluid balance. Suggestions for the resuscitation of elderly burn patients include noninvasive cardiac monitoring, the use of dobutamine if the patient has a low cardiac index, recognition that impaired cardiac function can lead to over-resuscitation, and the initiation of early hemofiltration when appropriate.[3]

Preventing Infection

Infection is the most significant cause of mortality in burn patients, with estimates ranging from 42% to 65% for mortality in burns associated with an infection.[21] Whether due to decreased immune function or long-term colonization by multidrug-resistant organisms, elderly patients are particularly susceptible. A 2016 study found that compared with younger controls, elderly burn patients showed a blunted early immune response to infection but a more robust late response.[22] Infection rates and sepsis in young versus elderly patients were not significantly different, but mortality was higher in older populations. Tissue samples showed a slower and later immune response in the elderly cohort, which could potentially leave such patients more susceptible to subsequent infection.[22]

Physiologic changes within the respiratory tract associated with aging—including decreased mucociliary clearance—may also contribute to an increased risk of respiratory infections.[23] Direct inhalation injury or prolonged intubation/tracheostomy further exacerbates the patients' susceptibility to respiratory complications. The additional damage to the airway (and cilia) means that these patients are less likely to clear sputum and adequately protect their airway. The increased stagnant sputum is known to lead to respiratory tract infections, further complicating the patients' hospital course.

Shared Decision-Making

Elderly patients have higher rates of frailty, comorbidities, decreased mobility, and poorer wound healing than similarly injured younger persons. Therefore, treatment options must balance the need to obtain wound closure to reduce illness or deformity with the added physiologic stress of operative interventions.

Previous studies of older adults engaged in decision-making around high-risk surgical procedures show that maintaining independence was a principal goal of any surgical therapy.[24,25] Other studies found few differences in quality of life or goals between younger and older burn patients.[26] Regardless, early and frequent goals of care discussions are essential as burns are a significant source of morbidity and mortality.

OPERATIVE MANAGEMENT OF BURNS IN THE ELDERLY
Acute Surgical Management in the Elderly

Since the 1970s, early excision and grafting have been the foundation of acute surgical burn care. Removing burn eschar decreases the risk of infection and improves length of stay and mortality.[27] In older adults, however, there has been a debate within the literature over the role of early excision and grafting. Studies from the 1980s and 1990s revealed that elderly patients did not benefit from the reduced length of stay and survival benefit of early excision and grafting that were seen in younger adults and pediatric patients.[28–30] Conversely, other studies—including prospective evaluations—from the same era found that early excision and grafting improved outcomes.[31,32] Yet the decision to pursue early excision and grafting is more likely to be determined by patient factors, including comorbidities and the ability to tolerate an operation. In their review of burns in older adults, Wibbenmeyer and colleagues found that delayed wound closure due to clinical instability or comorbidities was prevalent, and it was impossible to determine how this may have affected the overall survival rate.[33]

Fortunately, newer debridement modalities, including enzymatic debridement, may allow eschar removal outside an operating room, decreasing the patient's blood loss and physiologic stress. A recently published study of a bromelain-based debridement (Nexobrid, Mediwound Gmbh, Germany) demonstrated a more focused debridement, decreasing the overall wound requiring coverage.[34] In 2022, the US Food and Drug Administration approved bromelain-based debridement for adults with deep partial or full-thickness thermal burns. However, studies have brought into question whether enzymatic debridement is effective across all burn modalities, locations, and depths as it is not approved for chemical or electrical burns, or for burns on the face, perineum, or genitalia, or burns on the feet of patients with diabetes mellitus or the feet of patients with occlusive vascular disease, or circumferential burns, or burns in patients with significant cardiopulmonary disease, including inhalation injury.[35] Further investigation is needed to fully evaluate the utility of such products in persons with advanced age or frailty.

Wound Reconstruction in the Elderly

In their 2015 study on the pathophysiology of burns in the elderly, Jeschke and colleagues found that elderly burn patients had impaired wound healing compared with younger controls.[36] Specifically, elderly patients had impaired wound healing "associated with reduced stem cell pool, a diminished self-renewal capacity of progenitor cells, a deficient migration of mesenchymal stem cells, and an altered activation of essential signaling pathways for skin healing." The atrophic changes in the dermis and subcutaneous fat compounded the challenges of wound healing and of obtaining donor tissue via skin grafts or flaps.

The mainstay of autologous burn reconstruction is split-thickness skin grafts. Donor sites for split-thickness skin grafts have been shown to have longer healing times in older adults,[37] and locations may not be available for re-harvesting in cases where donor sites are limited.[38] Fortunately, newer technologies that expand donor cell availability (cultured epidermal autografts and spray-on skin cells) or biologic or synthetic skin substitutes may reduce the number of split-thickness donor sites needed to achieve coverage. However, these technologies are not universally available or may be prohibitively expensive. Similarly, synthetic or biologic skin substitutes may allow dermal replacement for wounds over vital structures or wounds that are not amenable to direct skin grafting (eg, tendons and bone). Further work is needed, particularly within the elderly population with poor donor site availability, to obtain cost-effective, widely available skin substitutes.

Data on advanced reconstruction in older adults, including free tissue transfer, are more prevalent within the oncologic literature (for head/neck and breast) than within the trauma or burn literature. However, both provide evidence of successful free tissue transfer in older patients. A recent systematic review and meta-analysis of head/neck and breast free tissue transfer in the elderly found a high success rate for flaps (95%) with no difference between the young and elderly patient groups regarding flap success rates or surgical complications.[39] However, the review found that systemic complication rates, preoperative American Society of Anesthesiology classification for risk, and mortality rates were higher among the elderly population. Other reviews of geriatric free tissue transfers have echoed sentiments that few differences in free flap outcomes exist between older and younger patients when the right flap is chosen for the right patient. In their review of 256 geriatric free flaps for any soft tissue defect (except autologous breast reconstruction), Wahmann and colleagues noted that their outcomes with geriatric patients were improved when they pursued axial flaps such as those of the rectus abdominis or latissimus dorsi. In contrast,

extremity-based flaps (such as the anterolateral thigh or gracilis flap) were more prone to atherosclerotic changes and complications.[40] The investigators also noted that while doing staged procedures involves multiple anesthesia events, some elderly patients seemed to benefit from staged vascular procedures to ensure adequate inflow to their reconstruction.

Data on free flaps within the burn literature are limited to case reports and series, often reflecting hand and extremity reconstruction with the occasional inclusion of elderly patients.[41,42] Regardless, high rates of microsurgical success can be achieved if preoperative optimization includes considering comorbidities, frailty, and the ability to participate in therapy and emphasizes the patient's reconstructive goals.[40]

The general principles of burn excision, coverage, and reconstruction (discussed in earlier articles) are the same for the elderly population. Clinicians must know the potential challenges of such care to make the best therapeutic decisions.

Burn Mortality in the Elderly: When Comfort Is the Best Treatment

With advances in critical care, there has been an overall improvement in elderly survival postburn.[43,44] However, burn or inhalation injury may exceed the patient's ability to recover. Significant inhalation injuries or large burns in the elderly carry high mortality and a substantial impact on future function and quality of life.[45] In these cases, further invasive treatments may be futile or simply against the overall goals of the patient and the patient's family. Palliative or comfort-driven care may be appropriate, and the involvement of a palliative care team can be very beneficial when available.

SUMMARY

With the rapid aging of the global population, clinicians treating burn patients must be aware of the unique challenges in this demographic. The physiologic changes of aging increase burn injury risk for elderly patients as well as make their recovery more difficult. Although the principles for resuscitation and wound management in the elderly are similar to those for younger patients, clinicians must understand the complications that are more prevalent in the older group. It is also imperative to consider the quality of life and palliative care needs of aged burn patients and engage with the patient and family about goals of care in order to best direct the therapy. More research is needed, particularly regarding frailty and its effects on burns. Efforts for the primary prevention of burn injury in this population are of utmost importance.

CLINICS CARE POINTS

- Burns in older adults have an overall low incidence but are still a significant cause of morbidity and mortality.
- Frailty is a better measure of physiologic reserve and outcomes than age.
- Have early talks with palliative care and rehabilitation services about the overall goals of care for elderly patients.
- Elderly patients may show a blunted initial immune response followed by a delayed response.
- Wound care and wound healing in elderly patients will follow a different timeline than in younger patients.

ACKNOWLEDGMENTS

The authors would like to thank Dave Primm of the UT Southwestern Department of Surgery for help in editing this article.

DISCLOSURE

The authors have no financial disclosures to state.

REFERENCES

1. World Health Organization (. Ageing and health. . Available at: https://www.who.int/news-room/fact-sheets/detail/ageing-and-health Web site. . Updated 2022. Accessed July 1, 2023.
2. Number of people 75 and older in the labor force is expected to grow 96.5 percent by 2030. Washington, DC: Bureau of Labor Statistics; 2021.
3. Jeschke MG, Phelan HA, Wolf S, et al. State of the science burn research: burns in the elderly. J Burn Care Res 2020;41(1):65–83.
4. Mendiratta P, Schoo C, Latif R. Clinical frailty scale. In: StatPearls. Treasure Island (FL): StatPearls Publishing LLC; 2023.
5. Masud D, Norton S, Smailes S, et al. The use of a frailty scoring system for burns in the elderly. Burns 2013;39(1):30–6.
6. Romanowski KS, Barsun A, Pamlieri TL, et al. Frailty score on admission predicts outcomes in elderly burn injury. J Burn Care Res 2015;36(1):1–6.
7. Curtis E, Romanowski K, Sen S, et al. Frailty score on admission predicts mortality and discharge disposition in elderly trauma patients over the age of 65 y. J Surg Res 2018;230:13–9.
8. Romanowski KS, Curtis E, Palmieri TL, et al. Frailty is associated with mortality in patients aged 50 years and older. J Burn Care Res 2018;39(5):703–7.
9. Galet C, Lawrence K, Lilienthal D, et al. Admission frailty score are associated with increased risk of acute respiratory failure and mortality in burn patients 50 and older. J Burn Care Res 2023;44(1):129–35.
10. Esechie A, Bhardwaj A, Masel T, et al. Neurocognitive sequela of burn injury in the elderly. J Clin Neurosci 2019;59:1–5.
11. Laiteerapong NHE. Chapter 16: diabetes in older adults. In: Cowie CC, Casagrande SS, Menke A, et al, editors. Diabetes in America. 3rd edition. Bethesda (MD): National Institute of Diabetes and Digestive and Kidney Diseases; 2018.
12. Romanowski KS, Sen S. Wound healing in older adults with severe burns: clinical treatment considerations and challenges. Burns Open 2022;6(2):57–64.
13. McGill V, Kowal-Vern A, Gamelli RL. Outcome for older burn patients. Arch Surg 2000;135(3):320–5.
14. Sen S, Romanowski K, Miotke S, et al. Burn prevention in the elderly: identifying age and gender differences in consumer products associated with burn injuries. J Burn Care Res 2021;42(1):14–7.
15. Wolff KB, Soncrant C, Mills PD, et al. Flash burns while on home oxygen therapy: Tracking trends and identifying areas for improvement. Am J Med Qual 2017;32(4):445–52.
16. Sharma G, Meena R, Goodwin JS, et al. Burn injury associated with home oxygen use in patients with chronic obstructive pulmonary disease. Mayo Clin Proc 2015;90(4):492–9.
17. American Burn Association. Position statement on home oxygen burn prevention. Available at: https://ameriburn.org/wp-content/uploads/2022/04/aba-home-o2-statement-final-3-8-22-2.pdf Web site. . Updated 2022. Accessed July 7, 2023.
18. Dong N, Gao N, Hu W, et al. Association of fluid management with mortality of sepsis patients with congestive heart failure: a retrospective cohort study. Front Med 2022;9:714384.
19. Boehm D, Menke H. A history of fluid management-from "one size fits all" to an individualized fluid therapy in burn resuscitation. Medicina 2021;57(2). https://doi.org/10.3390/medicina57020187.
20. Rizzo JA, Liu NT, Coates EC, et al. The battle of the titans-comparing resuscitation between five major burn centers using the burn navigator. J Burn Care Res 2023;44(2):446–51.
21. Savetamal A. Infection in elderly burn patients: what do we know? Surg Infect 2021;22(1):65–8.
22. Stanojcic M, Chen P, Xiu F, et al. Impaired immune response in elderly burn patients: new insights into the immune-senescence phenotype. Annals of surgery 2016;264(1):195–202.

23. Ho JC, Chan KN, Hu WH, et al. The effect of aging on nasal mucociliary clearance, beat frequency, and ultrastructure of respiratory cilia. Am J Respir Crit Care Med 2001;163(4):983–8.

24. Cooper Z, Courtwright A, Karlage A, et al. Pitfalls in communication that lead to nonbeneficial emergency surgery in elderly patients with serious illness: Description of the problem and elements of a solution. Ann Surg 2014;260(6):949–57.

25. Nabozny MJ, Kruser JM, Steffens NM, et al. Constructing high-stakes surgical decisions: It's better to die trying. Ann Surg 2016;263(1):64–70.

26. Santacreu E, Grossi L, Launois P, et al. The influence of age on quality of life after upper body burn. Burns 2019;45(3):554–9.

27. Janzekovic Z. A new concept in the early excision and immediate grafting of burns. J Trauma 1970; 10(12):1103–8.

28. Housinger T, Saffle J, Ward S, et al. Conservative approach to the elderly patient with burns. Am J Surg 1984;148(6):817–20.

29. Still JM, Law EJ, Belcher K, et al. A regional medical center's experience with burns of the elderly. J Burn Care Rehabil 1999;20(3):218–23.

30. Kirn DS, Luce EA. Early excision and grafting versus conservative management of burns in the elderly. Plast Reconstr Surg 1998;102(4):1013–7.

31. Kara M, Peters WJ, Douglas LG, et al. An early surgical approach to burns in the elderly. J Trauma 1990;30(4):430–2.

32. Deitch EA. A policy of early excision and grafting in elderly burn patients shortens the hospital stay and improves survival. Burns 1985;12(2):109–14.

33. Wibbenmeyer LA, Amelon MJ, Morgan LJ, et al. Predicting survival in an elderly burn patient population. Burns 2001;27(6):583–90.

34. Bernagozzi F, Orlandi C, Purpura V, et al. The enzymatic debridement for the treatment of burns of indeterminate depth. J Burn Care Res 2020;41(5): 1084–91.

35. Tapking C, Siegwart LC, Jost Y, et al. Enzymatic debridement in scalds is not as effective as in flame burns regarding additional eschar excision: a retrospective matched-control study. Burns 2022;48(5): 1149–54.

36. Jeschke MG, Patsouris D, Stanojcic M, et al. Pathophysiologic response to burns in the elderly. EBioMedicine 2015;2(10):1536–48.

37. Seppala T, Grunthal V, Koljonen V. Skin graft donor site healing among elderly patients with dermatoporosis - a case series. Int J Low Extrem Wounds 2022. https://doi.org/10.1177/15347346221087081. 15347346221087081.

38. Keck M, Lumenta DB, Andel H, et al. Burn treatment in the elderly. Burns 2009;35(8):1071–9.

39. Üstün GG, Aksu AE, Uzun H, et al. The systematic review and meta-analysis of free flap safety in the elderly patients. Microsurgery 2017;37(5):442–50.

40. Wähmann M, Wähmann M, Henn D, et al. Geriatric patients with free flap reconstruction: a comparative clinical analysis of 256 cases. J Reconstr Microsurg 2020;36(2):127–35.

41. Pan C, Chuang S, Yang J. Thirty-eight free fasciocutaneous flap transfers in acute burned-hand injuries. Burns 2007;33(2):230–5.

42. Abramson DL, Pribaz JJ, Orgill DP. The use of free tissue transfer in burn reconstruction. J Burn Care Rehabil 1996;17(5):402–8.

43. Pomahac B, Matros E, Semel M, et al. Predictors of survival and length of stay in burn patients older than 80 years of age: Does age really matter? J Burn Care Res 2006;27(3):265–9.

44. Lionelli GT, Pickus EJ, Beckum OK, et al. A three decade analysis of factors affecting burn mortality in the elderly. Burns 2005;31(8):958–63.

45. Mahar P, Wasiak J, Bailey M, et al. Clinical factors affecting mortality in elderly burn patients admitted to a burns service. Burns 2008;34(5):629–36.

Challenges in the Management of Large Burns

Hakan Orbay, MD, PhD[a], Alain C. Corcos, MD[b], Jenny A. Ziembicki, MD[b], Francesco M. Egro, MD, MSc, MRCS[a,b,*]

KEYWORDS

• Large burns • Mortality • Morbidity • Surgical care • Critical care • Palliative care

KEY POINTS

- Large burn injury presents unique challenges for the burn surgeon.
- Early excision and coverage of the large burns improve the survival.
- Alternative skin grafting methods and donor sites are valuable tools for the coverage of large burn wounds.
- Epidermal tissue engineering techniques have not reached the desired clinical potential but may be more efficient when combined with other techniques.
- Palliative care consultation should be considered early in the management of patients with large burns and poor prognosis.

INTRODUCTION

The improvements in critical care and resuscitation increased the survival rates of patients with large burns. However, infections, metabolic derangements, and coverage of these wounds continue to be a challenge. Immunosuppression makes these patients susceptible to invasive burn wound infections and hypermetabolic state increases the nutritional requirements. The best treatment for the burn infections is prevention via hygiene and isolation methods. Supportive care early in the management of these patients is imperative to get the patients ready for a series of surgical procedures for debridement and coverage of the burn wound. Split-thickness skin grafting (STSG) is the traditional coverage method for burn wounds but in case of large wounds may not be possible due to the lack of donor sites. Fortunately, a multitude of skin substitutes have been developed in recent decades to replace, temporarily or permanently, the autologous skin

and facilitate the coverage of the large burn wounds. Burn injury is not only a simple wound including the skin, but also a complex cascade of pathophysiologic events that should be addressed with vigilance for optimal outcomes.

BURN PATHOPHYSIOLOGY

The physiologic response to large burns is characterized by poor tissue perfusion due to profound capillary leakage and intravascular volume depletion, coagulopathy, and widespread release of inflammatory mediators.[1] These mediators act on T cells attenuating T-helper (Th)-1 response and enhancing the Th-2 and Th-17 responses.[2,3] This leads to an immunosuppressed state after large burns.[4]

Tumor necrosis factor (TNF)-α is an inflammatory mediator which is secreted primarily by macrophages and Th-1 cells. It is central to the systemic inflammatory response syndrome (SIRS) and sepsis seen in burn injuries.[5] Interleukin (IL)-6 is

[a] Department of Plastic Surgery, University of Pittsburgh Medical Center, Pittsburgh, PA, USA; [b] Department of Surgery, University of Pittsburgh Medical Center, Pittsburgh, PA, USA
* Corresponding author. Department of Plastic Surgery, University of Pittsburgh Medical Center, 1350 Locust Street, Medical Professional Building, Suite G103, Pittsburgh, PA 15219.
E-mail address: francescoegro@gmail.com

Clin Plastic Surg 51 (2024) 319–327
https://doi.org/10.1016/j.cps.2023.11.007
0094-1298/24/© 2023 Elsevier Inc. All rights reserved.

another inflammatory mediator that is elevated in the first week after burn injury.[6] IL-6 activates C-reactive protein.[7] IL-8 also peaks shortly after a burn injury and attracts neutrophils and granulocytes to the burn site.[8] High IL-8 levels correlate with increased mortality in large burns.[9] A similar correlation exists between the levels of granulocyte/macrophage colony-stimulating factor (GM-CSF) and monocyte chemoattractant protein-1 and mortality.[9] The levels of several other inflammatory cytokines are elevated soon after a large burn injury. These cytokines are IL-4, IL-2, IL-5, IL-7, IL-12 and its active form $P70$, IL-13, IL-17, and interferon-c.[5] Enzymes, matrix metalloproteinase (MMP)-8, and MMP-9 are released from neutrophils in response to increased levels of GM-CSF, IL-8, and TNF-α.[10] MMPs increase vascular permeability by breaking down the basement membrane in vessel walls and cause loss of intravascular volume and third spacing seen in burn injuries.[11]

Hypermetabolism

Hypermetabolism is a distinctive feature of systemic response to large burns. It occurs in conjunction with the SIRS as described above. Hypermetabolism increases mortality and may persists for up to 3 years after burn injury.[12] Hypermetabolic changes are seen primarily in the mitochondria of adipocytes. Increased amounts uncoupling protein-1 in mitochondria causes uncoupled mitochondrial respiration that is characterized by inner mitochondrial membrane proton conductance that proceeds without the presence of adenosine triphosphate (ATP) synthase. This derangement in mitochondrial function leads to heat production and shifts the metabolic function of adipose tissue from the storage of energy to the expenditure.[13,14] Skeletal muscle oxygen consumption increases due to increased ATP production.[15] Increase is also seen in ATP-consuming reactions required for protein synthesis, gluconeogenesis, and fatty acid cycling pathways.[16]

Central (hepatic) and peripheral (skeletal muscle) insulin resistance is a part of metabolic response to burn injury. It is probably due to a post-receptor defect involving the glycogen synthesis pathways.[17,18] Insulin resistance leads to hyperglycemia that promotes an aggressive hyperinflammatory response to burn injury.[19,20]

Coagulopathy

Coagulopathy in large burns is characterized by low levels of the anticoagulants: antithrombin, protein C, and protein S.[21] Protein C has potent anti-inflammatory and cytoprotective functions in addition to its anti-factor VIIIa function.[22] Activated form of protein C modulates the inflammatory response,[22] promotes angiogenesis[23] and stimulates reepithelialization.[24] The combined effect is the granulation tissue formation at the base of the wound, reduced inflammatory cell migration, and rapid epithelialization of the wound.[25,26] Inflammatory mediators TNF-α and IL-1 suppress protein C activation and expression, respectively.[27,28] The levels of both TNF-a and IL-1 increase immediately after a burn; therefore, the protein C levels decrease significantly in circulation. Protein C levels also differ significantly between survivors and non-survivors after large burns.[5]

CRITICAL CARE AND RESUSCITATION

Large cutaneous injury with or without concomitant inhalational injury presents several unique challenges to the burn surgeon. Inhalation injury can impact up to one-third of all major burn injuries and significantly increases mortality. Severe inhalation and cutaneous injury can have profound pathophysiologic consequences for the patient. Bronchoscopy should be performed to confirm inhalation injury in high-risk patients and vigorous chest physiotherapy, and ambulation should be initiated early once diagnosis is confirmed.[29] Nebulized N-acetylcysteine, salbutamol, and nebulized heparin can be used reduce the duration of mechanical ventilation after inhalational injury.[30]

Patents must be optimized hemodynamically and from a respiratory standpoint before undergoing operative intervention. High volume resuscitation secondary to capillary leak is often necessary resulting in increased skin turgor, pleural effusions, pulmonary edema, and infrequently, compartment syndrome. Parkland formula,[31] modified Brooke formula,[32] and the Rule of Tens[33] are the formulas used to calculate the amount of fluid needed in the first 24 hours following burn injury. Colloid and other rescue techniques should be used to avoid volume overloading during resuscitation.[34]

Intravenous access in large cutaneous burn patients may be complicated, and clean intravenous line insertion sites are often limited. Both peripheral and central venous insertion lines must be inspected and changed frequently as such patients are at high risk for bloodstream infections.[35] Large burn injuries demonstrate profound hypermetabolism, and early initiation of enteral feeds is essential. Every effort should be made to avoid interrupting feeds, which maybe continued throughout operative interventions. Monitoring of nutritional parameters is important, and consideration should be given to nutritional adjuncts such as oxandrolone and beta blockers (propranolol) to modulate the hypermetabolic response.[36]

TIMING OF SURGICAL INTERVENTION

After initial stabilization, surgical removal of the devitalized tissues (ie, eschar) down to a healthy well vascularized layer should be carried out early during hospitalization. Early debridement of the necrotic eschar reduces the inflammation and helps to reverse associated hypermetabolism and catabolism,[37] reduces mortality and length of hospital stay, and yields better functional and cosmetic outcomes.[38] It is often necessary in the patient with large burns to plan for serial surgical excisions, limiting the total body surface area (TBSA) excised. Operations should be limited in extent to avoid profound coagulopathy, acidosis, and hypothermia. Once recovered, patients may return quickly to the operating room until the excision is complete.

COVERAGE OF LARGE BURNS
Temporary Coverage

If the burn wound is not ready for coverage several temporary coverage methods can be used. These products help to prepare the wound for skin grafting and provide and additional layer of coverage, therefore increasing the stability of the final scar. There are numerous artificial dermal products in the market today and discussed in detail elsewhere in this volume.

Dehydrated human amniotic/chorion membrane
Sterilized, dehydrated human amnion/chorion membrane is composed of a single layer of epithelial cells, a basement membrane, and an avascular connective tissue matrix. Dehydrated human amniotic/chorion membrane (DHACM) contains growth factors that promote wound healing, including platelet-derived growth factor A and B, basic fibroblastic growth factor, and transforming growth factor beta 1. Amnion is used mainly for ophthalmologic burns.[39] It is available, readily, adherent, transparent (thus allowing wound monitoring), has the potential to reduce the risk of wound infection, and may have an analgesic effect. Disadvantages include difficulty in handling and fast degradation.[40]

Dermal replacement template
Dermal replacement template (DRT) is composed of a cross-linked bovine collagen and glycosaminoglycan dermal layer and a silicone epidermal layer.

Appropriate dressings are used to secure it in place and protect the wound area. The outer dressing can be changed as needed depending on the volume of exudate. Once the template has become vascularized (usually by 14 days), any silicone layer can be removed and an autograft applied.[41]

Acellular dermal matrix
Acellular dermal matrix is an allograft (also called homograft) product created from skin from a non-genetically identical deceased human donor that has been processed to remove the epidermis using a sequential decellularization process.[41] These decellularized matrices fully integrate into the wound bed after application, replacing lost dermal tissue and providing a scaffold into which the recipient's cells can grow and become vascularized, ultimately regenerating into normal skin.

Biodegradable temporizing matrix
Biodegradable Temporizing Matrix (BTM) is a fully synthetic product. It is applied in a two-stage approach. Given the potential protective nature of BTM against infectious complications and its ability to remain in place for longer periods without the need for delamination and application of STSG, BTM might prove to be beneficial in coverage of wound in those with extensively large percentage TBSA burns.[41,42]

Bilayered living cellular construct
The bilayered living cellular construct (BLCC) a dermal part (bovine type I collagen with human neonatal foreskin fibroblasts) and an epidermal part (keratinocytes). The BLCC template serves as a scaffold for neovascular and cellular infiltration from the wound bed. It can be used as a standard two-stage dermal template or as a single stage. In the two-stage procedure, the BLCC scaffold is gradually replaced with the patient's own collagen, forming a neo-dermis. After 2 to 3 weeks, the silicone epidermal layer is removed, and the wound is covered with a thin STSG.[41–43]

Xenografts
Skin xenografts (heterografts) are obtained from an unrelated species and can be used as temporary skin coverage, particularly for large burn wounds. Porcine grafts have been the most commonly used xenograft,[41] however, there's been research into the use of tilapia fish skin as xenograft.[41,43] They have been shown to decrease evaporative water loss, risk of infection, and encourage autologous epidermal growth.[42,43] However, xenografts do not revascularize; therefore, they do not last as long as allografts in the recipient bed.[41]

Cadaveric allograft skin

Cadaveric skin is often used for temporary coverage of large burns. It can provide wound coverage for up to 3 to 4 weeks.[43] When cryopreserved, allograft has an indefinite shelf life.[44] Limiting factors are availability of donors and high costs.[41]

The FDA-approved skin substitutes are summarized in **Table 1**.

Permanent Coverage

STSG is the current gold standard for the coverage of burn wounds. However, STSG is limited by donor skin availability especially in large burns. Moreover, the donor-site wound is associated with pain and additional scarring.[45]

Cultured epidermal autograft (CEA) was first described in 1975 as an alternative method for the coverage of large burns.[46,47] The promise of CEA is to provide large sheaths of skin grafts with minimal donor site requirements. A single full-thickness biopsy measuring 2 cm^2 can be expanded in area up to 10,000 times.[48] For patients with large burns, prompt skin coverage not only reduces the mortality but also is the key for acceptable functional and esthetic outcome.[49] As early excision became the standard of care for deep burns,[50] CEA generated great hopes for prompt reconstruction of the epidermal barrier in patients with large burns and limited donor sites. CEA can also be used to shorten the reepithelialization time of STSG donor sites (average of 7 days) allowing rapid reuse of these sites.[49] However, CEA faces many challenges in clinical application, such as low resistance to infection, long preparation time, high costs, and mechanical fragility.[51–53] The final take of CEA grafts can be as low as 16% because of the great fragility of the cultured keratinocyte sheaths.[49] Cuono method[54] combines the use of CEA with large-meshed STSG (1:6–1:12) for coverage of large burns. With this combined method, success rate can be as high as 85%[48,49,54] (**Fig. 1**). Younger age and low burned TBSA are also correlated with increased rates of CEA take.[48]

Meek's method was developed in 1958[55] and involved mechanical division of the skin graft into small pieces using a MEEK–Wall dermatome, followed by placement of these pieces onto the wound bed, dermal side facing down. Although it allows up to 10-fold skin expansion, this technique never gained widespread acceptance because it is labor-intensive and time-consuming.[56,57] There is a renewed interest in this technique with recent reports of success in patients with large burns.[58] Recent studies reported a graft take between 60% and 90% after an average of 2.21 surgeries.[57]

Other modified skin grafting techniques that have been described to overcome donor site limitations in patients with large burns are (1) Xpansion Micrografting System, (2) fractional skin harvesting, (3) epidermal suction blister grafting, and (4) ReCell technology.[45]

1. Xpansion Micrografting Technique: Based on a mincing device that STSG is passed through yielding 0.8 to 0.8 mm micrografts.

Table 1
FDA-approved skin substitutes used in burn coverage

Biobrane®	Biosynthetic dressing constructed of a silicon film and an embedded nylon fabric
Integra® DRT	Bovine, collagen/glycosaminoglycan dermal replacement
Ez Derm®	Aldehyde cross-linked porcine dermis
Epicel®	Autologous keratinocytes cultured ex vivo
OrCel™	Human dermal cells cultured in bovine collagen. Used for STSG donor sites in burn patients
TransCyte™	Human dermal fibroblasts grown on nylon mesh, combined with a synthetic epidermal layer
TheraSkin®	Cryopreserved split-thickness human skin allograft
AlloDerm®	Native human skin with intact basement membrane and cellular matrix
GraftJacket®	Acellular dermal regenerative tissue matrix
Helicoll (Encol)®	Acellular collagen matrix derived from bovine dermis
Kerecis™	Acellular dermal matrix derived from fish skin
Suprathel®	Synthetic membrane fabricated from a tripolymer of polylactide, trimethylene carbonate, and s-caprolactone

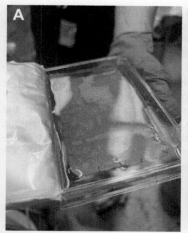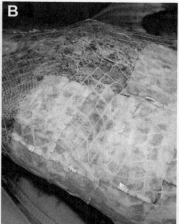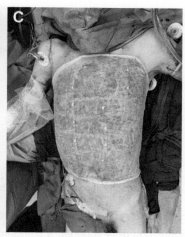

Fig. 1. The application of CEA to a patient with 48% TBSA burns after multiple rounds of cadaver grafting. (*A*) Cultured keratinocyte sheath in culture medium. (*B*) Application of CEA with STSG. (*C*) Final intraoperative result. (*Courtesy of* Francesco M. Egro, MD, Pittsburgh, PA.)

2. Fractional Skin Harvesting: Full-thickness microscopic skin tissue columns are harvested like fractional photothermolysis technique. The epidermis at the donor site heals within 24 hours with minimal scarring.
3. Epidermal Suction Blister Skin Grafting: The technique involves creation of an epidermal blisters using suction, which is then manually harvested from the donor site and transferred to the recipient site. A novel device called Cel-luTome (Kinetic Concepts, Inc, San Antonio, Texas) is available to harvest STSG using this method.
4. ReCell Technology: This technique involves enzymatic isolation of cells from the donor tissue and immediate autologous replantation to the wound without in vitro culture or expansion. The benefits of this method in terms of healing of burn wounds are controversial.[59]

In addition to the traditional STSG donor sites that might not be available in patients with large burns, soles of the feet, palm, scrotum, and scalp can be used as alternative donor sites for STSG.[60]

PALLIATIVE CARE

The survival of the patients with large burns has improved significantly since the adoption of early excision and grafting along with the advancement of critical care. However, patients with severe comorbidities and advanced age still have a poor prognosis and high mortality.[61] Baux score is a simple method predicting mortality after burn injury. It is calculated as: Percent Mortality = Age + Percent body burned.

Original Baux score was modified to include inhalation injury and recalibrated to reflect modern burn care results.[62,63] Prolonging the treatment of patients with high Baux scores and without a meaningful recovery is considered as "futile treatment."[64,65] Therefore, early involvement of a palliative care team should be considered in this cohort of patients.[64,66]

Palliative care is the "active holistic care of patients with advanced progressive illness" with a focus on minimizing illness-related discomfort and improving the quality of life for patients and their families.[65] Even though palliative care interventions can reduce health care utilization without increasing mortality for surgical patients, palliative care is still underused in burn patients due to misconceptions around it.[65,66]

Central components of palliative care include reducing the symptoms of disease, fostering communication, providing emotional and spiritual support to patients and families, and matching value-based goals with medical interventions.[66] Predicting survival in patients with large burns can be challenging due to the complex nature of physiologic changes associated with burn. This uncertainty complicates the goals of care/end-of-life care discussions. There is extensive literature regarding end-of-life care in elderly patients in medical intensive care units.[67,68] Burn units have a more heterogenous age distribution, with a larger population of younger patients, and unfortunately similar literature in burn patients is scarce.[69,70] Palliative care pathways, such as the Liverpool Care Pathway, are well established for palliation of patients in other settings but are rarely implemented in the patients with large burns.[71] As the patient population gets younger, a standardized protocol-based approach to end-of-life care discussions becomes more important. An example protocol for pediatric burn patients was published by Shriner's group.[72] Such protocols include triggers to initiate a palliative care consultation.

The early initiation of goals of care discussion in patients with large burns is appropriate and decreases the uncertainty surrounding the care of these complex patients. If the prognosis is poor, end-of-life care discussions, governed by the medical teams' clinical knowledge, should be initiated. The feelings, beliefs, and values of the patients' and their families should be taken into consideration during this discussion.[65] In general, patients with modified Baux scores between 120 and 150 are the best candidates for palliative care services, given the poor prognosis and unlikely survival. This group of patients might be best served by avoiding unnecessary interventions. The demographics of burn patients who are more likely to receive palliative care are summarized in **Box 1**.[73]

If at any point the decision to withdraw treatment is reached, appropriate comfort care measures should be implemented. A comfortable and dignified death relieves both the patient and family. A clear, standardized, and consistent documentation and communication are crucial during this transition process.[65]

SUMMARY

Early excision and coverage of the large burns improves the survival and prevents infections. However, it is important to understand and treat the complex pathophysiological derangements associated with large burn injury for a successful outcome. Nutrition and infection prevention are two main pillars of the supportive treatment. Skin coverage should be achieved as early as possible.

Alternative skin grafting methods and donor sites are valuable tools for this purpose. If the wound cannot be covered soon, temporary dressings and skin substitutes can provide a physiologic environment to facilitate wound healing and can be used as a bridge to definitive coverage. For patients with high Baux scores, palliative care consultation should be considered early in the hospital course. Palliative care is not synonymous with withdrawal of care. On the contrary, it improves the comfort of the patients and families during their often, lengthy hospital stay.

CLINICS CARE POINTS

- Large burns are not merely skin wounds; they trigger a complex pathophysiological response in human body. It is important to treat all aspects of burn injury for a successful outcome.
- Be comfortable with different coverage methods in case of donor site limitations.
- Pay attention to hypothermia and make every effort to minimize blood loss in the operating room.
- Palliative care is not same as withdrawal of care. Identify the patients who may benefit from palliative care early on.

DISCLOSURE

The authors have no disclosures.

REFERENCES

1. Guilabert P, Usúa G, Martín N, et al. Fluid resuscitation management in patients with burns: update. Br J Anaesth 2016;117(3):284–96.
2. Rani M, Zhang Q, Schwacha MG. Burn wound $\gamma\delta$ T-cells support a Th2 and Th17 immune response. J Burn Care Res 2014;35(1):46–53.
3. Sasaki JR, Zhang Q, Schwacha MG. Burn induces a Th-17 inflammatory response at the injury site. Burns 2011;37(4):646–51.
4. Zedler S, Bone RC, Baue AE, et al. T-cell reactivity and its predictive role in immunosuppression after burns. Crit Care Med 1999;27(1):66–72.
5. Lang TC, Zhao R, Kim A, et al. A critical update of the assessment and acute management of patients with severe burns. Adv Wound Care 2019;8(12):607–33.
6. Finnerty CC, Herndon DN, Przkora R, et al. Cytokine expression profile over time in severely burned pediatric patients. Shock 2006;26(1):13–9.

7. Jeschke MG, Finnerty CC, Kulp GA, et al. Can we use C-reactive protein levels to predict severe infection or sepsis in severely burned patients? Int J Burns Trauma 2013;3(3):137–43. Published 2013 Jul 8.

8. Kraft R, Herndon DN, Finnerty CC, et al. Predictive value of IL-8 for sepsis and severe infections after burn injury: a clinical study. Shock 2015;43(3): 222–7.

9. Finnerty CC, Jeschke MG, Qian WJ, et al. Determination of burn patient outcome by large-scale quantitative discovery proteomics. Crit Care Med 2013; 41(6):1421–34.

10. Pugin J, Widmer MC, Kossodo S, et al. Human neutrophils secrete gelatinase B in vitro and in vivo in response to endotoxin and proinflammatory mediators. Am J Respir Cell Mol Biol 1999;20(3):458–64.

11. Sternlicht MD, Werb Z. How matrix metalloproteinases regulate cell behavior. Annu Rev Cell Dev Biol 2001;17:463–516.

12. Jeschke MG, Gauglitz GG, Kulp GA, et al. Long-term persistence of the pathophysiologic response to severe burn injury. PLoS One 2011;6(7):e21245.

13. Patsouris D, Qi P, Abdullahi A, et al. Burn induces browning of the subcutaneous white adipose tissue in mice and humans. Cell Rep 2015;13(8):1538–44.

14. Sidossis LS, Porter C, Saraf MK, et al. Browning of subcutaneous white adipose tissue in humans after severe adrenergic stress. Cell Metab 2015;22(2): 219–27.

15. Biolo G, Fleming RY, Maggi SP, et al. Inverse regulation of protein turnover and amino acid transport in skeletal muscle of hypercatabolic patients. J Clin Endocrinol Metab 2002;87(7):3378–84.

16. Yu YM, Tompkins RG, Ryan CM, et al. The metabolic basis of the increase of the increase in energy expenditure in severely burned patients. JPEN J Parenter Enteral Nutr 1999;23(3):160–8.

17. Cree MG, Zwetsloot JJ, Herndon DN, et al. Insulin sensitivity and mitochondrial function are improved in children with burn injury during a randomized controlled trial of fenofibrate. Ann Surg 2007; 245(2):214–21.

18. Wolfe RR, Jahoor F, Herndon DN, et al. Isotopic evaluation of the metabolism of pyruvate and related substrates in normal adult volunteers and severely burned children: effect of dichloroacetate and glucose infusion. Surgery 1991;110(1):54–67.

19. Sun C, Sun L, Ma H, et al. The phenotype and functional alterations of macrophages in mice with hyperglycemia for long term. J Cell Physiol 2012;227(4): 1670–9.

20. Brauner H, Lüthje P, Grünler J, et al. Markers of innate immune activity in patients with type 1 and type 2 diabetes mellitus and the effect of the antioxidant coenzyme Q10 on inflammatory activity. Clin Exp Immunol 2014;177(2):478–82.

21. Lavrentieva A, Kontakiotis T, Bitzani M, et al. Early coagulation disorders after severe burn injury: impact on mortality. Intensive Care Med 2008; 34(4):700–6.

22. Mosnier LO, Zlokovic BV, Griffin JH. The cytoprotective protein C pathway. Blood 2007;109(8):3161–72.

23. Whitmont K, Fulcher G, Reid I, et al. Low circulating protein C levels are associated with lower leg ulcers in patients with diabetes. BioMed Res Int 2013;2013: 719570.

24. Whitmont K, McKelvey KJ, Fulcher G, et al. Treatment of chronic diabetic lower leg ulcers with activated protein C: a randomised placebo-controlled, double-blind pilot clinical trial. Int Wound J 2015; 12(4):422–7.

25. Jackson C, Whitmont K, Tritton S, et al. New therapeutic applications for the anticoagulant, activated protein C. Expert Opin Biol Ther 2008;8(8):1109–22.

26. Minhas N, Xue M, Fukudome K, et al. Activated protein C utilizes the angiopoietin/Tie2 axis to promote endothelial barrier function. FASEB J 2010;24(3): 873–81.

27. Nawroth PP, Stern DM. Modulation of endothelial cell hemostatic properties by tumor necrosis factor. J Exp Med 1986;163(3):740–5.

28. Yamamoto K, Shimokawa T, Kojima T, et al. Regulation of murine protein C gene expression in vivo: effects of tumor necrosis factor-alpha, interleukin-1, and transforming growth factor-beta. Thromb Haemost 1999;82(4):1297–301.

29. Enkhbaatar P, Pruitt BA Jr, Suman O, et al. Pathophysiology, research challenges, and clinical management of smoke inhalation injury. Lancet 2016; 388(10052):1437–46.

30. McGinn KA, Weigartz K, Lintner A, et al. Nebulized heparin with n-acetylcysteine and albuterol reduces duration of mechanical ventilation in patients with inhalation injury. J Pharm Pract 2019;32(2):163–6.

31. Pham TN, Cancio LC, Gibran NS, American Burn Association. American Burn Association practice guidelines burn shock resuscitation. J Burn Care Res 2008;29(1):257–66.

32. Haberal M, Sakallioglu Abali AE, Karakayali H. Fluid management in major burn injuries. Indian J Plast Surg 2010;43(Suppl):S29–36.

33. Chung KK, Salinas J, Renz EM, et al. Simple derivation of the initial fluid rate for the resuscitation of severely burned adult combat casualties: in silico validation of the rule of 10. J Trauma 2010; 69(Suppl 1):S49–54.

34. Orbegozo Cortés D, Gamarano Barros T, Njimi H, et al. Crystalloids versus colloids: exploring differences in fluid requirements by systematic review and meta-regression. Anesth Analg 2015;120(2): 389–402.

35. Younghwan C, Changmin S, Eunok P, et al. Use of blind placements of peripherally inserted central

catheters in burn patients: a retrospective analysis. Burns 2015;41(6):1281–5.

36. Ring J, Heinelt M, Sharma S, et al. Oxandrolone in the treatment of burn injuries: a systematic review and meta-analysis. J Burn Care Res 2020;41(1): 190–9.

37. Bakhtyar N, Sivayoganathan T, Jeschke MG. Therapeutic approaches to combatting hypermetabolism in severe burn injuries. J Int Critical Care 2015; 1(1):6.

38. Miroshnychenko A, Kim K, Rochwerg B, et al. Comparison of early surgical intervention to delayed surgical intervention for treatment of thermal burns in adults: a systematic review and meta-analysis. Burns Open 2021;5:67–77.

39. Lineen E, Namias N. Biologic dressing in burns. J Craniofac Surg 2008;19(4):923–8.

40. Fairbairn NG, Randolph MA, Redmond RW. The clinical applications of human amnion in plastic surgery. J Plast Reconstr Aesthet Surg 2014;67(5):662–75.

41. Haddad AG, Giatsidis G, Orgill DP, et al. Skin substitutes and bioscaffolds: temporary and permanent coverage. Clin Plast Surg 2017;44(3):627–34.

42. Song IC, Bromberg BE, Mohn MP, et al. Heterografts as biological dressings for large skin wounds. Surgery 1966;59(4):576–83.

43. Saffle JR. Closure of the excised burn wound: temporary skin substitutes. Clin Plast Surg 2009;36(4): 627–41.

44. Robb EC, Bechmann N, Plessinger RT, et al. Storage media and temperature maintain normal anatomy of cadaveric human skin for transplantation to full-thickness skin wounds. J Burn Care Rehabil 2001; 22(6):393–6.

45. Singh M, Nuutila K, Kruse C, et al. Challenging the conventional therapy: emerging skin graft techniques for wound healing. Plast Reconstr Surg 2015;136(4):524e–30e.

46. Rheinwald JG, Green H. Formation of a keratinizing epithelium in culture by a cloned cell line derived from a teratoma. Cell 1975;6(3):317–30.

47. Gallico GG 3rd, O'Connor NE, Compton CC, et al. Permanent coverage of large burn wounds with autologous cultured human epithelium. N Engl J Med 1984;311(7):448–51.

48. Homsombath B, Mullins RF, Brandigi C, et al. Application and management of cultured epidermal autografts on posterior burns-A 5-year, multicenter, retrospective review of outcomes. J Burn Care Res 2023;44(1):170–8.

49. Auxenfans C, Menet V, Catherine Z, et al. Cultured autologous keratinocytes in the treatment of large and deep burns: a retrospective study over 15 years. Burns 2015;41(1):71–9.

50. Herndon DN, Barrow RE, Rutan RL, et al. A comparison of conservative versus early excision.

Therapies in severely burned patients. Ann Surg 1989;209(5):547–53.

51. Clugston PA, Snelling CF, Macdonald IB, et al. Cultured epithelial autografts: three years of clinical experience with eighteen patients. J Burn Care Rehabil 1991;12(6):533–9.

52. Green H. Cultured cells for the treatment of disease. Sci Am 1991;265(5):96–102.

53. Ronfard V, Rives JM, Neveux Y, et al. Long-term regeneration of human epidermis on third degree burns transplanted with autologous cultured epithelium grown on a fibrin matrix. Transplantation 2000; 70(11):1588–98.

54. Cuono CB, Langdon R, Birchall N, et al. Composite autologous-allogeneic skin replacement: development and clinical application. Plast Reconstr Surg 1987;80(4):626–37.

55. MEEK CP. Successful microdermagrafting using the Meek-Wall microdermatome. Am J Surg 1958;96(4): 557–8.

56. Hsieh CS, Schuong JY, Huang WS, et al. Five years' experience of the modified Meek technique in the management of extensive burns. Burns 2008;34(3): 350–4.

57. Almodumeegh A, Heidekrueger PI, Ninkovic M, et al. The MEEK technique: 10-year experience at a tertiary burn centre. Int Wound J 2017;14(4): 601–5.

58. Lumenta DB, Kamolz LP, Frey M. Adult burn patients with more than 60% TBSA involved-Meek and other techniques to overcome restricted skin harvest availability–the Viennese Concept. J Burn Care Res 2009;30(2):231–42.

59. van Zuijlen P, Gardien K, Jaspers M, et al. Tissue engineering in burn scar reconstruction. Burns Trauma 2015;3:18.

60. Roodbergen DT, Vloemans AF, Rashaan ZM, et al. The scalp as a donor site for skin grafting in burns: retrospective study on complications. Burns Trauma 2016;4:20.

61. Jeschke MG, Pinto R, Kraft R, et al. Morbidity and survival probability in burn patients in modern burn care. Crit Care Med 2015;43(4):808–15.

62. Mrad MA, Al Qurashi AA, Shah Mardan QNM, et al. Risk models to predict mortality in burn patients: a systematic review and meta-analysis. Plast Reconstr Surg Glob Open 2022;10(12):e4694.

63. Osler T, Glance LG, Hosmer DW. Simplified estimates of the probability of death after burn injuries: extending and updating the Baux score. J Trauma 2010;68(3):690–7.

64. Pham TN, Otto A, Young SR, et al. Early withdrawal of life support in severe burn injury. J Burn Care Res 2012;33(1):130–5.

65. Ismail A, Long J, Moiemen N, et al. End of life decisions and care of the adult burn patient. Burns 2011; 37(2):288–93.

66. Madni TD, Nakonezny PA, Wolf SE, et al. The relationship between frailty and the subjective decision to conduct a goals of care discussion with burned elders. J Burn Care Res 2018;39(1):82–8.

67. Morgan J. End-of-life care in UK critical care units–a literature review. Nurs Crit Care 2008;13(3):152–61.

68. Zimmerman JE, Knaus WA, Sharpe SM, et al. The use and implications of do not resuscitate orders in intensive care units. JAMA 1986;255(3):351–6.

69. Fratianne RB, Brandt C, Yurko L, et al. When is enough enough? Ethical dilemmas on the burn unit. J Burn Care Rehabil 1992;13(5):600–4.

70. Wachtel TL, Frank HA, Nielsen JA. Comfort care: an alternative treatment programme for seriously burned patients. Burns Incl Therm Inj 1987;13(1):1–6.

71. Murphy D, Ellershaw J, Jack B, et al. The Liverpool care pathway for the rapid discharge home of the dying patient. J Integr Care Pathw 2004;8:127–8.

72. O'Mara MS, Chapyak D, Greenhalgh DG, et al. End of life in the pediatric burn patient. J Burn Care Res 2006;27(6):803–8.

73. Sheckter CC, Hung KS, Rochlin D, et al. Trends and inpatient outcomes for palliative care services in major burn patients: a 10-year analysis of the nationwide inpatient sample. Burns 2018;44(8):1903–9.

Moving?

Make sure your subscription moves with you!

To notify us of your new address, find your **Clinics Account Number** (located on your mailing label above your name), and contact customer service at:

Email: journalscustomerservice-usa@elsevier.com

800-654-2452 (subscribers in the U.S. & Canada)
314-447-8871 (subscribers outside of the U.S. & Canada)

Fax number: 314-447-8029

Elsevier Health Sciences Division
Subscription Customer Service
3251 Riverport Lane
Maryland Heights, MO 63043

ELSEVIER

Moving?

Make sure your subscription moves with you!

To notify us of your new address, find your Clinics Account Number (located on your mailing label above your name), and contact customer service at:

Email: journalscustomerservice-usa@elsevier.com

800-654-2452 (subscribers in the U.S. & Canada)
314-447-8871 (subscribers outside of the U.S. & Canada)

Fax number: 314-447-8029

Elsevier Health Sciences Division
Subscription Customer Service
3251 Riverport Lane
Maryland Heights, MO 63043

To ensure uninterrupted delivery of your subscription, please notify us at least 4 weeks in advance of move.

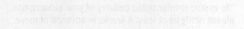